RESTORING
FISCAL SANITY
—— 2005 ——

ALICE M. RIVLIN *and* ISABEL SAWHILL
Editors

RESTORING
FISCAL SANITY
—— 2005 ——

Meeting the Long-Run Challenge

BROOKINGS INSTITUTION PRESS
Washington, D.C.

Copyright © 2005
THE BROOKINGS INSTITUTION
1775 Massachusetts Avenue, N.W., Washington, D.C. 20036
www.brookings.edu

Library of Congress Cataloging-in-Publication data are available

ISBN-13: 978-0-8157-7491-4
ISBN-10: 0-8157-7491-5

9 8 7 6 5 4 3 2 1

The paper used in this publication meets minimum requirements of the
American National Standard for Information Sciences—Permanence of Paper
for Printed Library Materials: ANSI Z39.48-1992.

Typeset in Sabon

Composition by Cynthia Stock
Silver Spring, Maryland

Printed by Victor Graphics
Baltimore, Maryland

This book is dedicated to

CHARLES L. SCHULTZE

our friend and colleague who has slain many a deficit dragon
and continues to be a source of wisdom and courage
on the issues addressed in this book.

Contents

Foreword

O
ne of the staples of American public debate is concern over the solvency of Social Security, the complexity of the tax code, the rising cost of health care, deficits in the federal budget, the nation's escalating debt to Asian central banks, and other perceived threats to our economic future. It is hard—but important—for citizens to evaluate the seriousness of these issues or the efficacy of the various proposals offered to solve them. This book is designed to help in that regard. It forecasts future pressures on the federal budget and offers a guide for judging the pros and cons of potential solutions and the political obstacles to their adoption.

At issue, both literally and figuratively, is the health of the country. Americans are living longer, and medical care is becoming both more effective and more expensive. The confluence of these two trends adds to the burden borne by the federal budget. Dealing with that growing problem will require Americans to make hard choices about what they want the federal government to do and how they want to pay for it. If current trends and policies continue, the cost of promises made to older people will require raising federal taxes to unprecedented levels or slashing other federal activities to levels not seen in the past half-century. These choices are complicated by the fact that the federal budget is already running a worrisome deficit that is projected to continue if policies are not changed.

Last year, in *Restoring Fiscal Sanity: How to Balance the Budget,* two Brookings economists, Alice Rivlin and Isabel Sawhill, assembled a team of experts who presented three options for reducing the deficit over the coming decade: one that emphasized spending cuts, one that relied on tax increases, and one based on a mixture of the other two. In this sequel, Alice and Belle have taken those options as a starting point to focus on the longer-run challenges posed by an aging population and escalating medical costs. It offers solutions that will have some appeal to those who believe government should do less, as well as to those who feel it should do more. It highlights the importance of thinking clearly about the size and role of government and of finding ways to overcome the political obstacles to taking action.

Despite its gimlet-eyed assessment of looming threats to the national well-being, this is not just a constructive piece of work but an essentially hopeful one. The authors believe that fiscal pressures provide an opportunity for needed reforms in the health care system, the federal tax code, and the Social Security system. These experts write from varying perspectives, but in the spirit of open-mindedness and collaboration that is crucial to the way we operate at Brookings; they have worked together to help the public understand the issues, using even their disagreements to illuminate the complexity of the trade-offs and policy challenges. Whatever their differences, the authors share a common objective of contributing to a civil and wide-ranging public dialogue and thus, ultimately, to better-informed political decisions.

STROBE TALBOTT
President

Washington, D.C.
April 2005

Acknowledgments

Brookings is grateful to the Annie E. Casey Foundation, the Charles Stewart Mott Foundation, and the Harry and Jeanette Weinberg Foundation for their continuing support of this project, but acknowledges that the findings and conclusions presented here are those of the authors alone and do not necessarily reflect the opinions of the foundations.

We also want to thank the members of our business advisory group, under the leadership of Geoffrey Boisi, for their support and advice. Advisory group members include Raymond Chambers, Richard Dumler, Fred Gluck, Thomas Healey, Robert Kaplan, Edward M. Lamont Jr., Robert Marks, Thomas Saunders III, and Roy Zuckerberg.

If the political system is going to take the kind of tough actions called for in this volume, members of the business community are going to need to make their voices heard, and we are extraordinarily grateful for the assistance of this group.

Many of the authors of this book participated in the first volume of this project and the editors thank them for their willingness to participate again this year, despite the many other demands on their time. These authors include Henry Aaron, William Gale, Ron Haskins, and Peter Orszag. The editors also thank the scholars who joined the group this year, including Jack Meyer, Rudolph Penner, John Shoven, and C. Eugene Steuerle.

Helpful advice on an earlier draft was received from Robert Bixby, James Capretta, Robert Greenstein, William Hoagland, Mark Prater, Robert Reischauer, and Allen Schick.

Special thanks are due to Daniel Klaff, Nathan Meath, and Steve Robblee for their research assistance; Anne Hardenbergh, Eileen Hughes, and Tanjam Jacobson for editing; Andrea Kane and Julie Clover for outreach; Eric Haven, Nathan Meath, and Steve Robblee for research verification; Larry Converse and Janet Walker for production of this volume; Evelyn Taylor for administrative assistance; and Anne Hardenbergh for coordinating the editing and production process.

Overview

Sometimes good news poses hard choices. Over the next several decades Americans will be forced to make difficult decisions necessitated by the good news that people are living longer and that medical care has become far more effective (albeit more expensive) than ever in history. These choices will require adjustments by almost everyone—families, communities, employers, and older people themselves—but they will be most starkly evident in the federal budget.

More than two-fifths of the federal budget is currently devoted to Social Security, Medicare, and Medicaid. Increased longevity, the retirement of the large baby boom generation, and rapidly increasing medical costs will drive spending on these programs sharply upward over the next three decades unless their current structure is radically changed (figure 1).

These projections dramatize that the current course is simply not sustainable.[1] Promises made to the elderly, especially about medical care, cannot be kept unless a way can be found to control or pay for the rise in health care costs. Even if medical costs grow more slowly, the cost of promises to seniors will force Americans to come to grips with very tough

Figure 1. *CBO Projection of Social Security, Medicare, and Medicaid Spending*

Percent of GDP

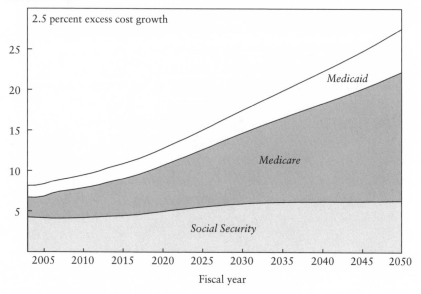

Fiscal year

Source: CBO, "The Long-Term Budget Outlook," December 2003.

budget choices. Unless taxes are raised to levels that are unprecedented in the United States, promises to the elderly will have to be dramatically pared back or other activities of the government will have to be slashed.

Much current debate focuses on the solvency of Social Security, but Medicare's fiscal problems dwarf the shortfalls in Social Security. Restoring long-run solvency to Social Security—whether by benefit cuts, revenue increases, or a combination of the two—would actually do relatively little to change the overall budget picture over the next several decades.

Although demographic and medical cost pressures will rise gradually over the coming quarter century, postponing action would be reckless and short-sighted. The sooner adjustments are made—whether in taxes or spending—the less drastic and disruptive they need to be. Moreover, responding to the longer-run imperatives is complicated by the fact that in fiscal year 2004 the federal government spent $412 billion (3.6 percent of GDP) more than it collected in revenues. These deficits are unlikely to decline substantially without changes in current policies.

Running an ongoing deficit of this magnitude is inappropriate in an economy that has recovered from recession and is growing at a healthy pace. Persistent deficits risk undermining the future growth of the economy, which will make it more difficult to deal with the demographic and medical cost pressures that loom ahead.

This book is designed to help the reader understand the dimensions of the budget problem, both in the near term and the longer run. Besides describing the problem, we offer a variety of concrete solutions. Some of these solutions will appeal to those who believe strongly in limited government. Others will appeal to those who favor expanding the government's role. Some will attract those who want to sort out what government does best from what it does less effectively. And some will appeal to those who are concerned about investing in children and in the future of the nation. Our objective is not to argue for one particular solution, but to demonstrate the magnitude and nature of the choices that will be required.

Budget Outlook for the Next Decade

As recently as fiscal year 2000 the federal budget was running a surplus of $236 billion, and was expected to stay in the black for the next decade or more. Then came the stock market crash, the recession of 2001 and the large tax cut that same year, the terrorist attacks on September 11, 2001, the wars in Afghanistan and Iraq, and the additional tax cuts in 2002 and 2003. By fiscal year 2004, the surplus had turned into a deficit equal to 3.6 percent of GDP. The most dramatic changes were on the revenue side. Federal revenues fell from 20.9 percent of GDP in 2000, the highest percentage since World War II, to 16.3 percent in 2004, the lowest percentage since 1959. Meanwhile, federal spending, which accounted for 18.4 percent of GDP in 2000, climbed to 19.8 percent in 2004.

A deficit of 3.6 percent of GDP would not be worrisome if it were expected to disappear as the economy grew faster, but, unfortunately, that is not the case. As detailed by Rudolph G. Penner and Alice M. Rivlin in

Figure 2. *Projected Deficit as a Percentage of GDP, 2004–15*

Deficit as percent of GDP

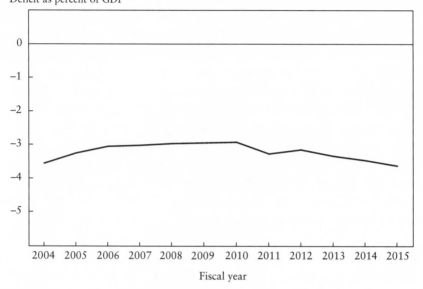

Fiscal year

Source: See adjusted baseline in table 1-1 on page 19.

chapter 1, projections based on reasonable assumptions show persisting deficits declining slightly in the next few years, but rising again toward the end of the ten-year period. Their projection for 2015 is a deficit of $715 billion, still around 3.6 percent of GDP (see figure 2).

Many people hope that economic growth will shrink or eliminate these deficits. Our projections are based on a 3.1 percent rate of real growth. Indeed, if the United States were lucky enough to enjoy a real growth rate of 4.3 percent over the coming decade—instead of the 3.1 percent assumed in our projection—the deficit would likely disappear by 2015.[2] However, rates of economic growth high enough to eliminate the deficits projected for the following decade (when aging and medical costs combine to increase spending) are not conceivable. Indeed, one of the surest ways to promote growth and improve future standards of living is to encourage national saving by reducing current borrowing by the federal government.

Deficits and National Saving

Deficits reduce national saving, which in turn reduces the income available to Americans in the future. The reduction in future income can come in two ways. In a relatively closed economy (one with few exports and imports) that is not in recession, large-scale government borrowing puts upward pressure on interest rates and other costs of capital. With investment more expensive, the economy will be deprived of the rapid growth of technology, equipment, and new skills that raise productivity and future incomes. But the U.S. economy is far from closed. In recent years, massive amounts of capital have flowed in from around the world, financing much of America's federal deficit, as well as its international (or current account) deficit, and mitigating any rise in interest rates that might have resulted from federal borrowing. This inflow of foreign capital has kept investment in the American economy strong, but it means that Americans are accumulating obligations to service these debts and repay foreigners out of their future income. As a result, the future income available to Americans will be lower than it would have been without the government deficits.

Foreign borrowing also makes the United States vulnerable to the changing whims of foreign investors. Opinions differ about how risky it is to rely on foreigners' continuing to purchase large portions of U.S. treasury bonds. Asian central banks, which are currently absorbing a large share of net U.S. treasury bonds issued, have a strong incentive to invest their growing reserves in dollar securities. This keeps their currencies from appreciating against the dollar and makes their exports attractive to Americans. This "co-dependency" could go on for years.[3] However, there is a risk that Asian central banks, or other large purchasers of dollar securities, will lose confidence in the ability of the United States to manage its fiscal affairs prudently and shift their purchases to euros or other currencies. Such a shift could precipitate a sharp fall in the value of the dollar, which could cause a spike in interest rates, a plunge in the stock and bond markets, and possibly a serious recession. The risk of such a fiscal meltdown is unknown, but it seems foolish to run this risk in order to perpetuate large federal deficits, which will ultimately reduce Americans' standard of living.

The aging of the population makes it especially urgent to increase national saving and grow the economy as quickly as possible. As the baby boomers retire and average longevity continues to increase, workers will be supporting a larger number of retirees unless working lives are extended and retirement deferred. There is no way to stockpile food, medical care, entertainment or other goods and services for use in a future year. The goods and services consumed by retirees, as well as by workers and their families, will all have to be produced in future years. The only way to increase that production is to increase national saving and invest that saving as productively as possible in knowledge, skills, and physical capital. This need to grow the future economy to accommodate more retirees means that proposals for reform of Social Security (see chapter 3), Medicare and Medicaid (chapter 4), and taxes (see chapter 5) should be judged in part by their contribution to increasing national saving.

Budget Outlook for the Longer Term

While the near-term budget picture shows a share of revenues that is low by historical standards and spending that is near the historical average, the picture changes quickly as the baby boom generation begins to retire. Longer-term budget projections are dominated by the spending pressures that flow from the combined effect of aging and the rising cost of medical care.

Social Security outlays are a relatively small part of the projected increase in spending associated with aging (see figure 1). Far larger increases in spending are expected in Medicare, as well as in Medicaid, which currently pays much more than half of the cost of long-term care for the elderly. How rapidly Medicare and Medicaid spending will rise depends, in turn, on the general rise in medical care costs. Past history is not encouraging because medical spending has been rising faster than the economy for decades. If medical care costs continue on their historic track (rising 2.5 percentage points faster than GDP), the increase in Medicare and Medicaid spending by 2030 will be more than four times the increase in Social Security spending. Even if medical care costs rise only 1 percentage point faster than GDP in the future, increased spending on

Medicare and Medicaid will be two-and-a-half times the Social Security increase between now and 2030.

The budget challenges from federally sponsored health programs are hard enough, but, as chapter 4 indicates, the nation faces an even larger challenge. Medicare and Medicaid are just part of the overall system of paying for health care. Successful modifications in Medicare and Medicaid will require reform of the entire health care system to rein in cost increases that threaten private as well as public budgets. Chapter 4 presents a menu of approaches to slowing the growth of health care spending. Unfortunately, the authors hold out little hope that the changes they examine will slow spending growth more than briefly. Many reforms might succeed temporarily, but acceptable steps are unlikely to have a large, sustained effect on the rate of growth in those outlays, which are driven primarily by new treatments and drugs that improve health and well-being.

Budget projections make clear that Americans face stark choices about what they want the federal government to do and how they want to pay for it. The long-run baseline projection we use, derived from the Congressional Budget Office (CBO), assumes that federal spending on all other programs (including defense) grows less rapidly than the economy and hence gradually falls as a percent of GDP, from about 10 percent at present to 7 percent in 2030 (table 1). Even with other spending declining, however, the projected spending increases in Social Security, Medicare, and Medicaid will drive federal spending to unprecedented levels. Total spending (less interest) would reach at least 24 percent of GDP in 2030 if medical costs continue their historic trend, and 21 percent if aggressive action succeeds in holding the increases to less than half the historic rate (table 1).

Revenues, in contrast, are not expected to grow commensurately. Over the past half century, federal revenues have averaged about 18 percent of GDP. When inflation, rapid economic growth or a booming stock market pushed revenues above 19 percent, tax rates were cut (for example, in 1981 and 2001), and the percentage dropped again. Hence even if revenues return to their historic average from their current low point, an unsustainable gap of about 6 percent of GDP (24 percent minus 18 percent) will remain between projected noninterest spending and revenues. Once interest payments on the debt are added to spending, the gap

Table 1. *Projected Federal Spending, 2030*[a]
Spending as a percent of GDP

Category	Current (2005)[b]	Base-line[c]	Smaller govern-ment[d]	Main-taining the Social Contract[e]	Investing in the Future[f]	Larger govern-ment[g]
Medicare and Medicaid[h]	4.2	11.5	5.7	11.5	8.4	11.5
Social Security[i]	4.2	5.9	5.5	5.9	5.7	5.9
Defense	3.8	2.8	2.0	2.0	2.8	2.8
Other federal spending[j]	6.2	4.3	2.9	2.4	6.1	5.8
Total primary spending	18.4	24.5	16.2	21.8	23.0	26.0
Interest spending[k]	1.5	2.0	2.0	2.0	2.0	2.0
Total spending	19.8	26.5	18.2	23.7	24.9	28.0

Note: See sources and notes to table 2-2 on page 41.

widens. The additional 2 percent of GDP shown in table 1 is premised on the optimistic assumption that the budget will be balanced over the coming decade. If balance is not achieved in this time frame, the gap will be still wider. Either way, Americans will have to choose whether they want to raise taxes enough to fill the gap between spending and revenues, drastically cut back on promises to the elderly, slash other activities of the federal government, or some combination of these approaches.

How does the gap between projected spending and the historical level of revenues translate into household incomes? In 2030, the average household will have an estimated mean income of $96,000 a year (in today's dollars) or 43 percent more than the $67,000 the average household had in 2005, assuming the economy grows at the rate projected by CBO. However, to pay for growing commitments to the elderly without decimating the rest of government or running large deficits, taxes would have to rise by more than 6 percentage points.[4] The average household's federal tax bill in 2030 would have to increase by about $7,000 relative to what it would have been with no growth in government. Fortunately, after-tax income would still rise from about $53,000 in 2005 to about $68,000 in 2030, or by 28 percent.[5] In short, households would be devoting some of their increased affluence to paying for a larger government and to eliminating current deficits. Alternatively, of course, they could choose a smaller government and a bigger increase in household incomes. Other choices are described below and summarized in table 1.

Short- and Long-Run Budget Choices

Last year, in *Restoring Fiscal Sanity: How to Balance the Budget*, we illus-trated three plans for achieving balance in the federal budget by 2014.[6] One was a "smaller government plan," which relied primarily on cuts in nondefense spending to achieve balance. One was a "larger government plan," which kept most current government programs, added moderate amounts of spending for health care, child care, and other programs favored by progressives, and required substantial tax increases to get to balance. One was a "better government plan," which reallocated federal spending, but kept it at about its current level. This plan achieved balance with less drastic spending cuts than the smaller government plan, and required a smaller revenue increase than the larger government plan. (Details can be found in last year's volume and in chapter 2.)

This year, we have applied a similar approach to the far more daunting problem of long-run budget choices (see chapter 2 by Alice M. Rivlin and Isabel Sawhill). Our smaller government scenario extrapolates the spend-ing cuts from last year's volume out to 2030 and dramatically restruc-tures the entitlement programs in a way that would require the elderly to pay for a much larger share of their own health and retirement expenses. The scenario assumes that most commercial and agricultural subsidies are eliminated; responsibility for education, housing, job training, the envi-ronment, and law enforcement is devolved to the states; real defense spending is kept below $400 billion; Social Security is indexed to prices instead of wages; and the rate of growth in health care costs is held equal to the rate of growth in the economy. Under this scenario, it is possible to reduce the size of government and provide modest additional tax cuts.

Our larger government scenario maintains current commitments to the elderly, provides for a more robust defense, and invests an additional 1.5 percent of GDP in a set of programs favored by many progressives. These investments include providing subsidized health care and child care for low- and moderate-income families, more access to higher education, universal pre-kindergarten programs for all children under age five with sliding-scale fees, additional wage supplements for low-income working parents, more funding for teacher training and other primary education needs, flexible grants to states for a variety of local needs, and a big boost in international aid to combat global poverty. However, investing in the future while simultaneously funding current promises to the elderly requires a hefty tax increase of 8 percentage points (from 18 to 26 percent of income).

Our two intermediate scenarios illustrate that holding tax increases to more moderate levels requires difficult choices. One scenario fulfills commitments to the elderly, but severely restricts other spending. The other scenario devotes resources to the kinds of investments contemplated in the larger government scenario, but still keeps tax burdens at a more reasonable level by restraining spending on the elderly. Options for achieving such restraint are presented in chapter 3 on Social Security and chapter 4 on health care.

Social Security

In chapter 3, Peter R. Orszag and John B. Shoven argue that there are no painless solutions to the projected imbalance in the Social Security system. Either benefits must be reduced or taxes increased. These two authors do not agree on the balance between the two choices or on the desirability of diverting some payroll tax revenues into private accounts. However, they agree that reforms should come sooner rather than later, that individual accounts will not by themselves solve the problem, that any reforms should be designed to increase national saving rather than rely on massive new borrowing by the federal government, that the elderly should be able to count on inflation-protected lifetime benefits that are not a dramatically reduced share of a worker's previous earnings, and that earnings for the most vulnerable (such as low-wage workers) should be protected. Orszag and Shoven present a menu of options for reform including increasing the retirement age, changing the benefit formula, and raising payroll taxes. Each of the authors favors a specific plan to achieve solvency and these plans are briefly described at the end of the chapter.

Health Care

Chapter 4, by Henry J. Aaron and Jack Meyer, provides more detail on the escalating cost of health care and the need to either curtail Medicare and Medicaid benefits sharply or raise taxes. In their view, neither a more efficient health care system nor reductions in spending on other government programs can plausibly fill the fiscal gap created by the rising cost of care. Moreover, unless the nation were to adopt lower standards of care for the elderly and others dependent on public programs, any changes in public programs would have to be part of a larger agenda that would revamp the health care payment system as a whole.

The authors emphasize the importance of multiple policy changes to improve efficiency and slow the growth of health care spending. Such measures could include greater use of computers to dispense medications and maintain patient records, well-designed malpractice reform, and greater market incentives for individuals and providers to be more selective in the kinds of treatments they choose to use. In addition, reforms of Medicare and Medicaid have some potential to reduce federal health care outlays. As examples, the authors discuss reforms that raise the age of eligibility for Medicare, require recipients to pay higher premiums, and encourage people to buy private long-term care insurance instead of relying on Medicaid to pay for nursing-home care. However, Aaron and Meyer believe these and other reforms discussed in their chapter will take years to implement and are unlikely to slow cost growth significantly even if they temporarily reduce the level of spending.

Revenues

The long-term fiscal gap could be reduced if the public were willing to pay more taxes, but increasing the level of revenues would put additional strain on a tax system whose structure is far from ideal. In chapter 5, William G. Gale and C. Eugene Steuerle address both the structure of the tax system and the need to align revenues with whatever level of spending is chosen. They argue that the tax system should be simpler, fairer, less intrusive, and more conducive to economic growth and efficiency. Gale and Steuerle discuss a variety of options, including replacing the current system with a consumption-based tax such as a national retail sales tax or a value-added tax. They also discuss reforms to the current system such as broadening the tax base by eliminating various deductions and exclusions, increasing incentives to save, fixing the alternative minimum tax, integrating corporate and individual taxes so that income is taxed only once, reducing the regressivity of the payroll tax, moving toward return-free filing, and providing the IRS with more resources for enforcement. All of these reforms are desirable regardless of the level of government spending, but tax burdens will obviously vary with the size of government. Under the smaller government scenario described in chapter 2, tax rates could be cut. But under all of the other scenarios, including those that trim spending, but are less draconian than the smaller government scenario, taxes would have to be raised. This could be achieved by allowing current tax cuts to expire, by aggressively reducing tax expenditures (deductions and exclusions), by introducing a value-added tax, or by pursuing some combination of these actions. For example, the larger government scenario could be paid for by introducing a 10 percent value-added tax, allowing the current tax cuts to expire, and closing a variety of tax loopholes.

The Opportunities These Budget Choices Create

Current public discussion of these challenges alternates between denial and alarm. Some of those in denial believe that faster economic growth will solve future budget problems painlessly. Others point out that projections are notoriously unreliable, and we can always hope for unexpected good fortune. Those who view the outlook with alarm, by contrast, sound as though the country were facing overwhelming disaster. They paint a picture so apocalyptic that solutions appear hopeless.

We believe both denial and panic are inappropriate and counterproductive. In the near term denial is risky, because sustained deficits will reduce the future income available to Americans and might precipitate a financial crisis. In the longer run denial is impossible. The aging population and the rising cost of medical care will certainly require changes in major federal entitlement programs or big increases in taxes or some combination of each. On the other hand, these challenges are not insurmountable. The United States is a rich, productive country with a flexible, adaptable economy. Moreover, the American population is not aging as fast as that of other industrial countries, such as Germany or Japan. In the United States, birth rates are higher, immigration is larger, and workers retire later.

Rhetoric that suggests the sky is falling impedes thinking about constructive solutions to problems that are, in fact, manageable. Indeed, these fiscal challenges can provide a much needed opportunity for reexamining and restructuring basic systems that are urgently in need of reform. The federal budget covers many programs that, once enacted, rarely get seriously reviewed. Some federal spending programs have outlived their usefulness, no longer address high priority needs, or foster inefficient activities. The relationship between the federal government and the states is affected by the accumulation of past actions made under other circumstances and in response to priorities that may have changed. (Some approaches to rethinking the federal role are considered in chapter 2.) Retirement and pension programs, both public and private, were created in an era when the labor force was growing much faster than the number of retirees and may no longer be appropriately structured for an aging society. (Social Security reforms are discussed in chapter 3.) Similarly, the way health care is delivered and paid for in the United States is a complicated patchwork of public and private mechanisms that favors high-cost care, results in extremely uneven standards, and leaves millions without health insurance coverage. Americans spend a larger fraction of their national resources on health care than other industrial countries, but have inferior health outcomes. (Health care policy options are discussed in chapter 4.) The federal tax code is also riddled with provisions that have accumulated over the years as Congress responded to current priorities or to the pleas of interest groups for tax relief. The result is a tax system that reduces economic growth by distorting economic choices, treats taxpayers in similar circumstances differently, and is widely perceived as both unfair and inordinately complex. (Tax reform is addressed in chapter 5.)

In short, each of these systems is a messy, incoherent accumulation of past incremental policies that would greatly benefit from rethinking and restructuring. Whether the American political system can face up to this challenge is another matter. As emphasized by Isabel Sawhill and Ron Haskins in chapter 6, making progress on reducing deficits or on restructuring entitlements or taxes has always been difficult, and appears to be especially difficult in the current political environment. Past agreements that have produced such progress, such as the Social Security reforms of 1983, the tax reforms of 1986, and the budget bills enacted in 1990, 1993, and 1997, have depended for success in varying degrees on presidential leadership, bipartisan support, a high degree of public concern, the use of outside commissions or other unorthodox processes to provide political cover for elected officials, and rules that have helped these officials to maintain fiscal discipline. Interviews conducted for this book with twenty Washington insiders from both parties, all of whom have participated in past negotiations on these fiscal matters, suggested two conclusions. The first is that without presidential leadership, an aroused public, and bipartisan support, major change is highly unlikely. The second is that the unwillingness of the majority party to put taxes on the table, or to cut spending in any major way, is impeding current progress. For these reasons, serious deficit reduction is unlikely to occur unless a perceived crisis forces the public and its representatives to rethink entrenched positions.

In our view, neither major party alone can resolve these challenges. Solutions will require ideological flexibility and a degree of bipartisan cooperation that has not been seen in recent years. For example, it is unrealistic to think the federal budget can be balanced either entirely by cutting spending or entirely by raising taxes. The necessary spending cuts would be unacceptable to many in both parties, and so would the necessary tax hikes. As in the 1990s, bringing currently projected deficits under control will require a series of bipartisan legislative packages involving a mix of spending cuts and revenue increases, reinforced by healthy growth in the economy. Similarly, reducing medical cost increases will entail increased reliance on market forces, which Republicans favor, combined with some government regulation (say, of pharmaceutical prices) more acceptable to Democrats. And if Republicans want to introduce private accounts into Social Security, they will have to give the Democrats something they want in return, such as allowing some current tax cuts to expire.

In the rest of this book we explore options for resolving the fiscal challenges facing Americans, and the opportunities for reform they present. Where we have preferences we do not hide them. Our main objective, however, is to show that solutions are possible and to stimulate dialogue that can lead to workable, bipartisan solutions.

Notes

1. Three publications from non-partisan government sources were used as the basis for projections throughout the volume. "The Budget and Economic Outlook: Fiscal Years 2006 to 2015," published by the Congressional Budget Office in January 2005, provided the initial baseline estimates for 2005 and the subsequent ten-year period. (The authors of this volume adjusted the CBO baseline based on likely changes to current law.) Another CBO report, "The Long-Term Outlook," published in December 2003, was used as the basis for cost estimates for the four spending scenarios in 2030 that are found in chapter 2. The "2004 Annual Report of the Board of Trustees of the Federal Old-Age and Survivors Insurance and Disability Insurance Trust Funds," published in March 2004, provided many of the projections about Social Security's financial status and also was used to estimate growth in Medicare costs due to changes in life expectancy.

2. Authors' calculation based on the Congressional Budget Office's 0.1 percent "rule of thumb" growth sensitivity analysis. See Congressional Budget Office, "The Budget and Economic Outlook: Fiscal Years 2006 to 2015," January 2005, Appendix A.

3. Catherine L. Mann, "Managing Exchange Rates: Achievement of Global Re-balancing or Evidence of Global Co-dependency?" *Business Economics,* July 2004, 20–29.

4. Specifically, they would have to increase by 7.2 percentage points. The difference reflects the fact that GDP is about 20 percent higher than personal income. The primary reason for the difference is depreciation, which is a nontaxable expense to businesses.

5. At 18 percent of GDP, taxes are roughly $14,000 per household ($0.18 \times 1.2 \times \$67,000$) and after-tax income is $53,000, on average. By 2030, taxes would need to be about $28,000 ($0.24 \times 1.2 \times \$96,000$) and after-tax income would be $68,000 under the maintaining the social contract scenario. With no growth in government, taxes would need to be about $21,000 ($0.18 \times 1.2 \times \$96,000$) in 2030 and after-tax income would be $75,000.

6. Alice M. Rivlin and Isabel Sawhill, eds. *Restoring Fiscal Sanity: How to Balance the Budget* (Brookings, 2004).

1

Dimensions of the Budget Problem

RUDOLPH G. PENNER AND
ALICE M. RIVLIN

The nation is headed for a fiscal train wreck. Unless entitlement growth is curbed or tax burdens are raised to unprecedented levels, exploding deficits will threaten economic stability—probably within two decades. In the shorter run the deficit outlook is not as dire, but deficits are large enough to have a corrosive impact on economic growth. Moreover, it would be beneficial to keep the public debt as low as possible, to provide flexibility as budget problems grow in the future.

An aging population and rapidly rising medical costs will lead to budget problems in the future. Social Security, Medicare, and Medicaid will be most affected, and to the extent that their growth is left unchecked, other government programs may be squeezed out of the budget. In confronting this problem, Americans will be forced to make basic choices about what they want their federal government to do and how they want to pay for it. In the process, they will also have the opportunity to redesign some basic building blocks of public policy, such as the federal tax code, the health care payment system, and the division of responsibilities between the federal government and the states.

In this chapter we describe the dimensions of the budget dilemma facing the administration and Congress, both over the next decade and over the longer run. We explain the risks posed by escalating deficits and the benefits of addressing budget issues sooner rather than later. We argue that the budget choices facing Americans are manageable, especially if the country acts quickly, but hard choices are inescapable. Over the next several decades, the fundamental question is how Americans will react to growing budgetary pressures. Will they choose to maintain the benefits promised to the elderly without cutting other activities of the federal government significantly? If so, will they be willing to pay commensurately higher taxes? Or will they pare back benefits for older people and shift more responsibilities onto the states and the private sector, in order to avoid higher taxes at the federal level? These options are explored in greater detail in subsequent chapters.

The Budget Outlook: The Next Ten Years

Although the future is always uncertain and all projections are hazardous, any informed discussion of budget choices must start with projections of what is likely to happen to the budget if current policies are continued. Our starting point is the most recent baseline projection of the Congressional Budget Office (CBO). That baseline is too optimistic, however, because the CBO is forced by law to assume that discretionary spending is frozen in real terms and that current tax law is extended. Current tax law implies, among other things, that recent tax cuts will be allowed to expire. We therefore used an "adjusted" baseline that assumes that nondefense real discretionary spending grows with the population; that defense spending is consistent with continued outlays on Iraq, Afghanistan, and the war on terrorism; and that the tax cuts now in place will be extended—as strongly recommended by President Bush (table 1-1). The adjusted baseline also assumes that the alternative minimum tax will not be allowed to affect a rapidly growing proportion of income taxpayers. [1]

As may be seen in figure 1-1, the official CBO baseline shows the deficit declining from $412 billion (3.6 percent of gross domestic product)

Table 1-1. CBO Baseline and Adjusted Baseline, 2004–15[a]
Billions of dollars

Item	2004	2005	2006	2007	2008	2009	2010	2011	2012	2013	2014	2015
CBO baseline												
Spending												
Defense	454	464	438	435	447	457	468	484	488	504	516	529
Appropriated	441	466	476	485	493	502	511	523	534	546	559	572
Mandatory	1,237	1,317	1,380	1,450	1,529	1,620	1,713	1,824	1,896	2,028	2,159	2,303
Subtotal (excluding interest)	2,132	2,248	2,294	2,369	2,469	2,580	2,693	2,830	2,918	3,078	3,234	3,403
Net interest	160	178	213	249	274	289	303	311	314	311	308	303
Total	2,292	2,425	2,507	2,618	2,743	2,869	2,996	3,142	3,232	3,389	3,542	3,706
Revenue	1,880	2,057	2,212	2,357	2,508	2,662	2,806	3,062	3,303	3,474	3,657	3,847
Deficit or surplus	**-412**	**-368**	**-295**	**-261**	**-235**	**-207**	**-189**	**-80**	**71**	**85**	**115**	**141**
Adjusted baseline												
Spending												
Defense	454	494	512	518	536	554	572	594	605	629	650	672
Appropriated	441	466	481	494	507	520	534	551	568	586	604	623
Mandatory	1,237	1,317	1,380	1,450	1,529	1,620	1,713	1,824	1,896	2,028	2,159	2,303
Subtotal (excluding interest)	2,132	2,278	2,373	2,461	2,572	2,694	2,819	2,969	3,069	3,243	3,413	3,597
Net	160	178	216	259	292	319	345	372	401	431	464	499
Total	2,292	2,456	2,589	2,720	2,864	3,013	3,164	3,341	3,470	3,674	3,877	4,096
Revenue	1,880	2,056	2,194	2,307	2,438	2,568	2,701	2,799	2,925	3,070	3,222	3,381
Deficit or surplus	**-412**	**-399**	**-395**	**-413**	**-427**	**-445**	**-463**	**-542**	**-545**	**-604**	**-655**	**-715**

Source: Authors' calculations; Congressional Budget Office (CBO), "The Budget and Economic Outlook: Fiscal Years 2006 to 2015" (Washington, January 2005); and William G. Gale and Peter R. Orszag, "The Outlook for Fiscal Policy," *Tax Notes*, February 14, 2005, pp. 841–54.

a. The adjusted baseline modifies the CBO baseline to extend expiring tax provisions, adjust the alternative minimum tax, and keep per capita discretionary spending constant, and includes supplementary spending on Iraq, Afghanistan, and the war on terrorism derived by inflating the CBO's estimated peak cost by inflation and population growth.

Figure 1-1. *Baseline and Adjusted Outcomes as a Percentage of GDP, 2004–15*

Percent of GDP

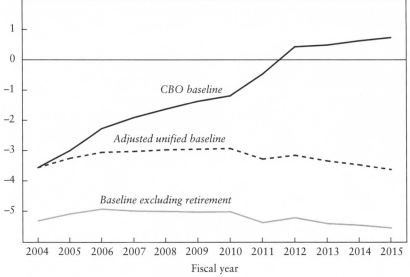

Fiscal year

Source: CBO, "The Budget and Economic Outlook: Fiscal Years 2006 to 2015."

in fiscal year 2004 and turning into a surplus of $141 billion by fiscal year 2015. However, the adjusted baseline makes the deficit picture look far less rosy. The difference is primarily due to the assumed extension of the large tax cuts enacted in 2001 and 2003. In the adjusted budget, the unified deficit (including Social Security and Medicare) declines in dollar terms early in the period, but rises again toward the end of the period because of the extended tax cuts. The estimated unified budget deficit for 2015 is $715 billion, or about 3.6 percent of GDP in that year. In other words, the unified deficit in the adjusted baseline is about the same size in relation to the economy in 2015 as in 2004. Moreover, the unified budget projections give a misleadingly optimistic view of the deficit over the next decade, because temporary surpluses in the Social Security and Medicare trust funds offset the deficits in the rest of the budget. If these temporary surpluses in the retirement programs were pulled out of the budget, the deficit in 2015 would rise to $1,093 billion, or about 5.6 percent of GDP.

President Bush's budget recommendations for fiscal 2006 show much lower deficits in the short and medium term than those in our alternative baseline. He proposes severe restraints on domestic discretionary spending, similar to those he recommended for 2005 for all domestic spending outside homeland security. For that year, Congress pretty much accepted his recommendations for total domestic spending; if it does so again for 2006 and there are no domestic supplemental appropriations, the discretionary spending path will be somewhat lower than is assumed in our alternative scenario. The president would also like to reform the alternative minimum tax in a way that is "revenue neutral," although revenue neutrality has not been precisely defined.

In addition to the proposals contained in his budget, the president has proposed a reform of Social Security that would divert payroll taxes into personal accounts. Although much of this diversion would have to be paid back by the account holder over the very long run, it would significantly increase the unified budget deficit for several decades.

It is not clear how successful the president will be in pursuing his budget and Social Security goals, and it is even more uncertain what will happen once he leaves office. If the president fails to sell his Social Security reform but is even moderately successful in convincing Congress to implement his spending reductions, the deficit is likely to be lower than in our alternative path. Nevertheless, if the tax cuts are extended, our alternative path is still likely to be closer to reality than is the CBO baseline. The economic and technical assumptions underlying both paths could, of course, turn out to be wrong in either direction.

Current deficits, and those projected for the coming decade, do not reflect historically high rates of federal spending. As may be seen in figure 1-2, federal spending has varied over the years, but has averaged about 20 percent of GDP, approximately its current share. Federal revenues have also varied, averaging about 18 percent of GDP.[2] As the result of tax cuts and the end of the stock market boom of the 1990s, revenues had fallen to 16.3 percent of GDP for 2004—the lowest share since 1959—and they are not expected to rise appreciably faster than the economy over the decade.

Figure 1-2. *Total Revenue and Outlays as a Percentage of GDP,*
1962–2015

Percent of GDP

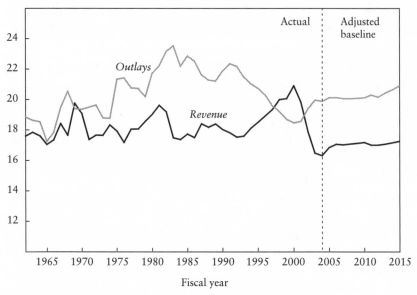

Source: See figure 1-1.

Short-Run Risks to Economic Growth and Stability

Although deficits helped to stimulate the economy as it recovered from
the recession that began in 2001, there is strong consensus among economists that large continuing deficits are inappropriate when, as now, the
economy is growing at a healthy clip and approaching full employment.
There is considerable controversy, however, about whether deficits of the
range projected for the coming decade should be a major cause for alarm.
The question is whether the damage such deficits might do in the next few
years is worth the pain inherent in closing them by raising taxes and
reducing spending.

Those who are most concerned about deficits—including the authors
of this chapter—focus on the facts that federal deficits reduce national

saving, make the United States increasingly dependent on the willingness of foreigners to hold increasing quantities of U.S. Treasury bonds, and load the cost of current federal spending onto future taxpayers. Private saving in the United States has declined over a long period and is considerably lower than that in most industrial countries. When private domestic saving is low, large scale increases in public debt certainly put some upward pressure on interest rates. It may not take a very large increase in interest rates to discourage investment or make housing more expensive. But focusing on the interest rate effect misses the most important impact of deficits. Whatever the effect on interest rates, deficits will reduce national wealth in the long run by absorbing scarce private saving and increase our liabilities to foreigners by sucking in foreign investment. Lower national wealth implies lower investment in new factories and equipment, which in turn slows productivity growth and reduces future standards of living. A higher foreign debt implies that more of our national product has to be devoted to servicing that debt. And a higher domestic public debt implies that government has to devote more of its tax revenues to paying interest on government bonds and has less revenue left to pay for public services.

In recent years, the willingness of public and private investors to buy and hold large quantities of American securities has allowed the American economy to live beyond its means. Even through the 2001 recession and its aftermath, huge amounts of money have flowed into the United States to finance both private investment and public borrowing. In particular, Asian central banks have chosen to hold large fractions of their growing reserves in U.S. Treasury bonds. Part of their motivation has been to protect their own countries' exports by preventing the appreciation of their currencies with respect to the dollar. The big uncertainty now is how long the rest of the world, especially Asian central banks, will continue to be willing to buy the U.S. Treasury bonds that finance our federal deficit. Recent declines in the value of the dollar, especially with respect to the euro and the pound, suggest that foreign investors, including Asian central banks, may be becoming less sanguine about holding increasing quantities of dollar-denominated assets.

Those who argue that projected deficits are manageable point out that the recovering U.S. economy is still an attractive place for global investors to put money, and U.S. Treasuries continue to be rated the safest securities in the world. They regard the recent decline of the dollar as a normal correction that will stimulate U.S. exports, control imports, and reduce the current account deficit, not a danger sign for the future.

However, there is no denying that the continuous U.S. government borrowing of more than 3 percent of GDP to finance current federal spending makes the United States vulnerable to changes in perceptions of U.S. fiscal responsibility and of the future value of the dollar. If those perceptions turn negative, they could become self-fulfilling. Currency markets often overshoot. A sharp plunge in the value of the dollar could trigger a flight from dollar securities (including U.S. Treasuries), a spike in interest rates, and possibly a serious recession. Even if the chance of such a financial meltdown is low, it is foolish to take the risk. It is especially foolish when known demographic pressures dictate that the need to attract foreign capital to finance U.S. deficits will grow, not diminish, after the end of the ten-year window.

In sum, while the United States might be able to continue running deficits in the projected range (between 3 and 4 percent of GDP) for some years without financial catastrophe, no one can be sure. Such a policy makes us vulnerable to the whims of international investors and passes the burden of paying for current government services to future federal taxpayers, whose burdens will also be increased by the aging of the population and rising medical costs.

Demography, Health Costs, and the Budget

Domestic federal spending is, in large part, driven by demographics. Almost one-half of nondefense spending outside interest goes to people aged sixty-five and over.[3] Social Security and Medicare are the most important elderly programs, by far. (They also serve the disabled, and Social Security provides for survivors.) Nevertheless, heavy spending on the aged can be found throughout the budget—in long-term care expenditures by Medicaid, in civilian and military retirement programs, and in welfare programs such as Supplementary Security Income. Thus the aging of the population combined with soaring health costs will create severe budget pressures for the foreseeable future. Although this issue is often associated with the aging of the baby boom generation, whose members will begin applying for Social Security in 2008, continued increases in life expectancy are quantitatively more important in the very long run. The impact of aging on the budget will not disappear when the last baby boomer passes from the scene.

The average age of the population is also increasing because the number of young people is growing so slowly. The baby boomers did not produce enough potential taxpayers to support them well in their old age, and the immigration of younger workers, while growing rapidly, has not increased enough to make up the labor force shortfall. The growth in the number of retirees would not present a serious problem were it not for the slowing growth of the labor force. Of course, only a budget wonk would emphasize the bad news in all this. The really good news is that more and more people are leading longer and healthier lives.

Long-Run Budget Scenarios

The fact that such a large share of federal spending is devoted to programs for the elderly, especially the health care of the elderly, guarantees enormous upward pressure on federal spending over the next several decades. Long-run spending scenarios published by the Congressional Budget Office in 2003 dramatize this point. In its most pessimistic scenario, the CBO assumes that per capita medical care costs will rise 2.5 percent faster a year than GDP over the foreseeable future. This is the rate of excess growth experienced over the period 1960–2001. Under this assumption, spending for Social Security, Medicare, and Medicaid would rise from about 8 percent of GDP at present to 11 percent in 2015 and 17 percent in 2030.

As shown by figure 1-3, spending for Medicare and Medicaid dominates federal spending projections. Projected increases in Social Security spending seem relatively minor in comparison. Even if the Social Security benefits promised in current law are paid over the whole period, Social Security outlays are only expected to rise from 4 percent to 6 percent of GDP between 2005 and 2030. In fact, between 2030 and 2050, Social

Figure 1-3. *Historical and Projected Components of Federal Spending,*
1962–2050

Percent of GDP

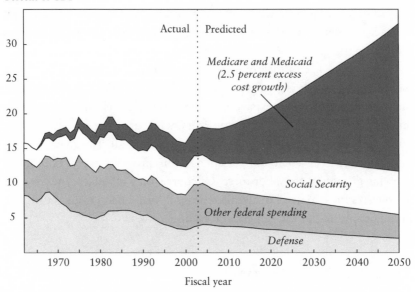

Fiscal year

Source: CBO, "The Long-Term Budget Outlook" (Washington, December 2003).

Security outlays come close to stabilizing relative to GDP, rising only
about 0.4 percent of GDP over those two decades.

The assumption that excess health cost growth exceeds 2.5 percent a
year is more pessimistic than that used by the trustees of the Medicare
system. They assume that excess growth eventually slows to 1 percent per
year. This assumption is, however, based more on a hope than a promise.
There is no indication that health cost growth will slow in the future,
except that health costs will take up an implausibly large share of the
GDP if there is no deceleration. As shown in the figure 1-4, the difference
in assumptions has a large impact on long-run budget projections. With
2.5 percent excess growth, Medicare and Medicaid spending will absorb
11.5 percent of the GDP by 2030. With 1 percent excess growth, "only"
8.4 percent of GDP will be absorbed. This result dramatizes the crucial
importance of making an extraordinary effort to reduce the historic rate
of health care spending increase (see chapter 4).

Figure 1-4. *Total Federal Spending for Medicare and Medicaid under Different Excess Cost Growth Assumptions*

Percent of GDP

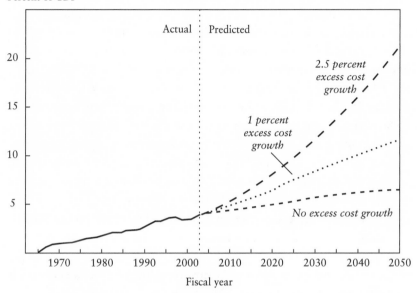

Source: See figure 1-3.

The CBO projects that the rest of federal spending (that is, total federal spending less Medicare, Medicaid, and Social Security) will actually decline as a share of GDP over the next several decades. Indeed, even in its highest spending scenario, the rest of federal spending (excluding interest) declines from 10.0 percent of GDP in 2003 to 8.2 percent in 2030 and 7.5 percent in 2050.[4] The decline occurs primarily because defense spending is assumed to stabilize eventually at a constant real level. One wonders whether a constant real level of defense spending is plausible, given that it would most probably imply a gradual decline in force levels, which may not prove feasible unless the world becomes substantially less threatening in the future.

Combining the CBO's long-run spending scenarios with assumptions about future revenues illustrates the magnitude of the fiscal train wreck implicit in the combination of aging and rapidly growing heath costs. Suppose that the overall tax burden is allowed to drift upward until it reaches the average of the last thirty years—18.4 percent of GDP. When this revenue assumption is combined with the CBO's most pessimistic spending path (the one that assumes that excess health spending will remain at its historic rate of 2.5 percent above GDP), deficits skyrocket and the nation's public debt grows at an accelerating rate. The implied ratio of debt to GDP, 37 percent in 2004, reaches 100 percent by 2027. Even when excess spending is restrained to 1 percent above GDP growth, the debt still grows at an accelerating rate and it reaches 100 percent of GDP by 2037. A debt explosion is avoided only when there is assumed to be no excess health cost growth. Given past history, it is hard to imagine this outcome without a radical reform of our entire health care system.

In a debt explosion, much of the problem is caused by the interest charges required to service projected debt. As debt starts to grow rapidly, interest charges grow faster than annual revenues. There is a powerful compounding effect as the government is forced to borrow more to cover a growing interest bill, and that in turn causes the interest bill to grow at an ever faster rate. The various CBO scenarios illustrate that the timing of the consequent debt explosion is sensitive to relatively small changes in spending and tax assumptions. Nevertheless, a calamity occurs in all cases. It is like the difference between falling off a twenty- and a sixty-story building: the end result is the same, even though it takes longer to get there if the building is taller. It is important to emphasize that absent reform, a financial collapse is likely to occur long before the Social Security trust fund is expected to be unable to pay current benefits (around 2042). In other words, we face an overall budget problem, not just a trust fund problem.

Dealing with Past Entitlement Growth

In reflecting on the challenges involved in dealing with a 6 to 9 percent increase in the cost of Social Security, Medicare, and Medicaid relative to GDP by 2030, it is useful to look back over the past fifty years and ask how growth in these programs was dealt with previously. Fifty years ago, Medicare and Medicaid had not been invented and Social Security outlays absorbed only a tiny portion of GDP. Now, the three programs absorb over 8 percent of GDP. However we dealt with this growth, it did not seem too painful. Can't we do the same thing again?

We did not deal with past growth by raising taxes. Indeed, the 2004 tax burden, at 16.3 percent of GDP, is almost identical to that in 1951. More generally, the tax burden has been remarkably constant, with significant tax cuts following whenever the tax burden has crept above 19 percent of GDP. It is more difficult to say how much of the burden was financed by an upward trend in the budget deficit, because the deficit tends to be highly erratic. However, the deficit today is less than 4 percent of GDP, and though they were smaller than today's, deficits were not unknown in the 1950s. Therefore, it would be hard to argue that as much of one-half of the growth was financed by the deficit's upward trend.[5]

By far the most important source of financing for the growth in Social Security, Medicare, and Medicaid has been a secular downward trend in defense spending. Defense accounted for about 10 percent of GDP after the Korean War; today it is only about 4 percent of GDP, despite wars in Iraq and Afghanistan. In the CBO's scenarios the decline continues, but even this projected decline, which we suspect is highly optimistic, is not nearly sufficient to finance future growth in spending for the elderly.

The overwhelming conclusion is that the United States cannot deal with future budget pressures using past practices. The alternatives are clear: tax burdens will have to be raised far beyond the levels experienced in the past (and that will probably require a substantial tax reform); or programs for the elderly and other health programs will have to be radically reformed; or the rest of government will have to be squeezed to almost nothing; or deficits will reach intolerable levels.

The Response of Financial Markets

Should the budget follow any of the disaster scenarios just described, it is interesting to ask when international financial markets would become alarmed. Would they wait until a debt explosion was under way, or would they be impressed when an explosion began to show up in the CBO's ten-year budget projections? If the latter, financial markets could become unstable in the next decade. But there are already many projections of a debt explosion. Why are financial markets so sanguine, and why is U.S. sovereign debt given the highest possible rating by debt rating services?

There are two possible explanations. Either investors have great confidence in the United States' ability to reform, or they do not believe the projections.[6] The latter would not be surprising, since five-year estimates of the budget imbalance implied by constant policies have an average error of over 3 percent of GDP—almost $450 billion at 2009 levels of GDP. One can see why markets may be skeptical about twenty-five-year forecasts when economists have grave difficulty getting it right for much shorter periods. But our fear of a financial calamity is based to a considerable degree on demographic projections that are unlikely to be wildly wrong—certainly not wrong enough to obviate the conclusion that the present situation is unsustainable.

The Accuracy of Long-Run Projections

In fact, long-run forecasts of Social Security spending tend to be highly accurate. Social Security policies have been quite stable over the past twenty years, and almost all the people that will be drawing benefits over the next thirty years have already been born. The annual forecasts for the benefit-to-GDP ratio in 2000 made by the Social Security trustees from 1985 varied over a range of less than 0.7 percent of GDP. One reason that estimates of benefits relative to GDP are so accurate is that initial benefits are indexed to wages. Hence, overestimates of GDP growth tend to be accompanied by overestimates of benefit growth, and underestimates of GDP growth by underestimates of wages.

Admittedly, forecasts of health costs are much less accurate, and errors in this area are often a major source of error in short-run forecasts of the budget balance. But although the health cost forecasts used in the above analysis may be quite wrong, it is less likely that they err on the side of pessimism. The most pessimistic spending path assumes that excess cost growth will equal the average over the previous forty years. There is no reason to think that the rate of innovation and technical change in health care has slowed. It is very difficult to argue that the assumed spending paths are overly gloomy, especially when the health cost assumptions are combined with the CBO's modest path for defense spending.

False Promises

Although the vast majority of budget analysts agree that current budget policy is unsustainable, there are a few dissenters who would argue that our analysis is far too pessimistic. For example, some argue that the U.S. economy can grow its way out of the problem if marginal tax rates are kept low and regulation unobtrusive. We do not think that this is a plausible argument. While there is no doubt that good tax and regulatory policies can enhance growth, the effects would have to be unbelievably large to solve the problem. Increased growth would reduce the Social Security problem only marginally. The problem is that initial benefits are indexed to wages. Faster wage growth causes faster benefit growth, and so the promises become more expensive as the economy grows more quickly. Faster growth helps a little, in that the benefit computation is not indexed to wage growth after age sixty, and benefits grow only at the rate of price increases after retirement. But it is impossible to imagine growth fast enough to completely solve the Social Security problem.

The relationship between economic growth and the Medicare and Medicaid problem is somewhat more complex, but no more reassuring. We believe that faster growth would increase the demand for health services because the standard of living would increase. Increased demand is likely to increase excess cost growth, not reduce it.

Other observers have suggested that the answer lies in increased immigration. There is no doubt that immigrants play an important beneficial role in the U.S. economy. Without immigration and high birth rates among recent immigrants, the labor force would be declining in the long run and the country's demographic problems would begin to resemble the much more severe problems faced by Europe and Japan. But immigrants grow old, too. Unless immigration constantly grows relative to the size of the labor force—and we find this politically implausible—it cannot help much in the very long run.

The Importance of Acting Quickly

There are three major reasons for acting quickly. First, necessary benefit reductions can be phased in more gradually, thus providing an early warning for those approaching retirement. Future retirees can then plan to save more or work longer. The increase in the full retirement age implemented for Social Security in 1983 was a model for providing ample warning. It was phased in so slowly that it did not affect anyone over the age of forty-five. If future benefit reductions are to play a significant role in stabilizing the long-run fiscal outlook, they will have to start relatively soon. Unfortunately, it is already too late to provide the seventeen-year warning contained in the 1983 reform.

If action is taken early, it is also easier to maintain the average real Social Security benefit enjoyed when the reform is implemented. The decision to index initial benefits to wages in the late 1970s reflected the philosophy that benefit growth should keep pace with wage growth, that is to say, the replacement rate for retirees should be kept constant automatically. As a result, current law implies almost a 40 percent increase in the average real benefit between 2003 and 2030. But today's payroll tax structure, together with today's surplus, are sufficient to finance an increase of about 8 percent in the average real Social Security benefit between 2003 and 2030.

The political debate is really about how much to let the replacement rate erode over time. Advocates of the current system want relatively minor reductions, whereas others would let the replacement rate erode substantially, perhaps replacing traditional benefits with individual accounts (see chapter 3 for an elaboration of this debate). Abstracting from the controversial issue of individual accounts, a political debate over how much to raise benefits as living standards increase should be much less painful than a debate over how much to cut real benefits. Unfortunately, there is not much time left to talk. Average real benefits are being increased every year, and the financial condition of the system is growing worse. If we wait until after 2010 to reform, it will no longer be possible to maintain real benefits through 2030 without raising payroll taxes.

A third reason for acting quickly is to reduce the level of the national debt. With a lower debt, the burden imposed by interest costs can be lowered substantially, because interest cost savings compound quickly. If the growth rate of revenues were increased by 0.1 percent a year starting in 2004, the revenue increase in 2015 would be $35 billion, but all else equal, the indirect interest saving would be $10 billion that year. In other words, the indirect interest effect, or "bonus," amounts to 28 percent of the direct effect of the tax increase.[7]

Lower deficits would also bring a higher rate of economic growth. But the benefits of growth are not so straightforward. We have already noted that faster economic growth does not much reduce the burden imposed by Social Security, Medicare, and Medicaid. Still, one might expect people to be less resistant to tax increases and cuts in promised benefits as living standards rise. Unfortunately, history shows no sign of that. As already noted, federal tax burdens have remained remarkably constant since World War II as living standards have soared. And while Social Security benefit growth was cut in 1977 and in 1983, it was because the system was under financial duress, not because people were willing to give up benefits as living standards rose.[8] Indeed, Congress and the president have just added massively to the generosity of Medicare by passing a prescription drug program in 2003.

Conclusions

The budget numbers are bleak. Few deny that current fiscal policies are unsustainable. Yet, reform should not be as hard as it seems to be. As budget problems grow, society will be becoming ever more affluent. The debate will be about how to use that growing affluence, not about how to impoverish either the elderly or nonelderly population. Some may not wish to tolerate significantly higher taxes to support the most affluent portions of the population in ever longer retirements. Others may feel that considerably higher tax burdens are justified to maintain something close to the present system. There is much room for compromise between these extreme positions. However, one cannot argue that Americans can maintain today's benefit structure while continuing to enjoy tax burdens lower than the average of the last thirty years.

Notes

1. Our adjusted baseline is based on the analysis of William Gale and Peter Orszag, modified to include continued defense spending on Iraq, Afghanistan, and the war on terror (see table 1-1). William G. Gale and Peter R. Orszag. "The Outlook for Fiscal Policy," *Tax Notes,* February 14, 2005, pp. 841–54.

2. Congressional Budget Office averages 1962 to 2004. CBO, "The Budget and Economic Outlook: Fiscal Years 2006 to 2015" (Washington, January 2005), historical tables F-2.

3. CBO, *Federal Spending on the Elderly and Children* (Washington, June 2000).

4. Calculations exclude Medicare offsets from "the rest of government" percentages.

5. Rudolph G. Penner, *Errors in Budget Forecasting* (Washington: Urban Institute, 2001).

6. Sentiments about the ability to reform can be found in reports on the creditworthiness of the U.S. government. For more details, see Rudolph G. Penner, "The Financial Consequences of Fiscal Paralysis," *National Budget Issues* 2 (Washington: Urban Institute, June 2004).

7. Calculations are based on the adjusted baseline in table 1-1.

8. In 1983 the Social Security trust fund had no more assets. In 1977 the system was not in as much trouble; that year's reform corrected a flaw in indexing that caused benefits to rise faster than intended as inflation rose. Left uncorrected, it would have created severe financial problems in a very few years.

2

The Size and Role of Government

ALICE M. RIVLIN AND
ISABEL SAWHILL

A mericans face serious budget choices over the coming decade and
far more daunting ones afterward. This chapter first examines
three illustrative plans for achieving balance in the unified budget over
the next ten years and then turns to the options for meeting the larger,
longer-term challenge: how to balance the budget as the population ages
and medical care grows more effective and more expensive. As the baby
boom generation retires, average life spans continue to increase, and
medical costs continue to rise, federal spending will accelerate rapidly
unless current policy changes drastically. There are only three choices.
Americans can reduce existing government commitments to the elderly,
slash other government programs, or accept higher taxes.

Current Federal Spending

Federal spending in 2004 is projected to be $2.3 trillion, or about 20 per-
cent of GDP. Social Security, Medicare, and Medicaid together make up

We are deeply indebted to Daniel Klaff and Nathan Meath for their extensive
assistance with this chapter.

Figure 2-1. *Federal Spending, 2004*

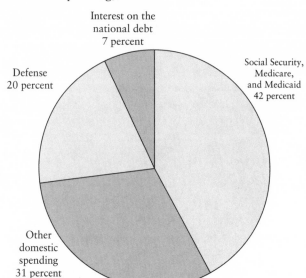

Source: Congressional Budget Office, "The Budget and Economic Outlook: Fiscal Years 2006 to 2015" (January 2005).

42 percent of total federal spending (figure 2-1).[1] These big programs, which benefit primarily the elderly, will drive increases in federal spending over the longer run, but they reflect only a small part of what the federal government does. National defense, international affairs, homeland security, law enforcement, education, scientific research, public lands and the environment, veterans' affairs, agriculture, welfare, child care, job training, and a host of other program areas make up the rest of government.

National defense accounts for 20 percent of total federal spending, and domestic spending outside of the big three entitlement programs accounts for 31 percent (figure 2-1). Within domestic spending, "discretionary spending," which is appropriated annually, accounts for about 19 percent of all federal spending and "mandated" programs, which are not subject to annual appropriation, account for about 12 percent. It is not realistic to attempt to shrink the deficit by focusing on any one of those categories of spending alone. For example, balancing the budget in 2015 by cutting domestic discretionary spending alone would require cutting each program 86 percent in 2015, or virtually closing down the government.[2] Cuts of that magnitude in, say, national parks, federal prisons, or education of children with special needs would outrage the public, and few politicians would remain in office if they supported such cuts. Moreover, defense spending is already close to historic lows relative to the size of the economy, and cutting it is especially difficult in wartime. Domestic mandatory programs include agricultural subsidies, veterans' benefits, and other programs with strong political support. Social Security, Medicare, and Medicaid present a tempting target for budget-cutters because they are so large and are likely to grow rapidly if no changes are made. Chapters 3 and 4 explore the potential for reducing the growth of these programs. However, achieving substantial savings in entitlements over the next decade would necessitate immediate cuts that have been ruled out of bounds by most politicians because they would threaten the well-being of those who currently are retired or near retirement. In sum, there is no quick or easy way to curb government spending. Raising taxes is equally difficult.

Budgetary Options for the Next Decade

Last year, in *Restoring Fiscal Sanity: How to Balance the Budget*, we illustrated the tough choices required to reach budget balance over the next decade. We described three deficit-reduction packages, each of which was designed to achieve balance in the unified budget by 2014 but reflected different views about the size and role of government. Given last year's projections, meeting this goal required finding $534 billion in spending reductions or revenue increases by 2014. Interest saved by reducing the debt over the period would contribute another $153 billion in that year, to close a total gap of $687 billion.[3]

The "smaller government plan" illustrated choices that would appeal to those who believe that the federal government does too much, especially in the domestic arena, and that the budget should be balanced primarily by reducing spending. This plan cut federal expenditures as a share of GDP from 20.2 percent in 2003 to 18.3 percent in 2014. To accomplish

the reduction, we focused on federal programs that have been identified
by conservatives as candidates for elimination, privatization, or devolution to state and local governments. We cut $400 billion from projected
expenditures in 2014 by eliminating commercial and agricultural subsidies ($138 billion); devolving all responsibility for education, housing,
job training, the environment, and law enforcement to the states ($123
billion); reducing wasteful spending ($7 billion); and slowing the growth
of other domestic spending ($58 billion) as well as the growth of the big
three entitlements, Social Security, Medicare, and Medicaid ($74 billion).[4]
Commercial subsidies include farm price supports and grants for energy
research and development; airports and air traffic control; community
development; the Agency for International Development; and the Export-
Import Bank, which provides services to companies that do business
abroad. Eliminating all of the grants to state and local governments for
education, housing, job training, the environment, and law enforcement
would force those levels of government to cut back services, deliver them
more efficiently, or raise their own taxes. Other major savings in the
smaller government plan came from reducing funding for the space program and for health research, raising the Social Security retirement age in
2012, changing the way cost of living increases are calculated, and
increasing premiums for Medicare recipients.

The process of selecting programs to be cut in the smaller government
plan made clear that reducing the size of the federal government by even
a couple of percentage points of GDP requires extremely painful political
choices. Those choices would have major impacts on state and local governments and the private sector. Many of the programs cut in the smaller
government plan have powerful political support among voters and their
elected representatives. Moreover, even though we ignored the political
consequences, we were unable to reach balance in 2014 with spending
reductions alone and had to resort to revenue increases to attain that goal.

The "larger government plan," by contrast, was designed to appeal to
those who believe that the federal government is not doing enough to
improve education, help people pay for health care, or support low-
income working families. In crafting this plan, we left most federal
domestic activities intact, made modest cuts in defense spending, and

allowed some additional spending for health, education, and other domestic priorities favored by most Democrats. We financed the additional spending and balanced the budget by rolling back recent tax reductions for high-income taxpayers and adding a new national consumption tax. By the end of the period, total federal spending as a share of GDP climbed to 20.9 percent, from 20.2 percent in 2003.

We also described a "better government plan," designed to keep the size of government roughly at its current level but to reallocate spending to improve government performance. It included a mix of spending cuts and tax increases as well as a major reallocation of spending toward high-priority areas, including international assistance to fight global poverty and spur economic development in regions of the world that have become seedbeds for terrorism. Also included was funding to make the homeland more secure, restructure the safety net to encourage and reward work, improve preschool programs for children, extend health care coverage to lower-income families, and help states fund the No Child Left Behind Act of 2001. Funding these priorities *and* eliminating the deficit required a combination of tax increases and steep cuts in other spending for everything from farm subsidies to manned space flight, but the cuts were not as drastic as the ones included in the smaller government plan.

Table 2-1 summarizes the amount of deficit reduction accomplished by each plan and the different ways in which balance was achieved in each case. The table was taken from last year's book, and greater detail on each of the plans can be found in that volume.

Not much has changed since last year. Our projected deficit for 2015 is only slightly higher than it was in 2014 ($715 billion versus $687 billion), the result of a number of offsetting changes. Revenues are a little higher but so are spending and interest on the debt.[5]

Long-Term Scenarios

For about fifty years, Americans have acted as though they wanted to prevent total federal spending from rising to much more than 20 percent of GDP.[6] At the end of the cold war, when defense spending fell as a percent

Table 2-1. *Three Plans to Balance the Budget by 2014*
Billions of dollars

Change	Better government plan	Larger government plan	Smaller government plan
Total deficit reduction	687	687	687
Interest payment change	–153	–153	–153
Revenue change	401	629	134
Programmatic spending net change	–134	95	–400
Defense net change	–60	–60	0
Increase	0	0	0
Decrease	–60	–60	0
Nondefense net change	–74	155	–400
Increase	41	185	0
Decrease	–115	–30	–400

Source: Alice M. Rivlin and Isabel Sawhill, eds., *Restoring Fiscal Sanity: How to Balance the Budget* (Brookings, 2004).

of GDP, domestic spending—especially Medicare, Medicaid, and Social Security—rose to keep total spending at approximately 20 percent of GDP.

But in coming decades Americans will face a new situation. The combined impact of the baby boomers' retirement, increased longevity, and more effective but more expensive medical care will push federal spending (less interest) to almost 25 percent of GDP by 2030. The stark reality is that if Americans honor their current promises to older people without reducing other federal responsibilities, they will have to increase the federal spending share of GDP by at least 6 percent and add that much to their tax bill. If they choose to keep the federal share close to its historic 20 percent, they will have to choose between substantially reducing the benefits promised to older people and drastically cutting back on projected spending for other federal programs. Many of those programs (education, transportation, and scientific research) are investments in younger people and the future growth of the economy. Those decisions will be made gradually and many compromises are possible, but basic choices must and will be made.

We have constructed four budget scenarios for 2030 that illustrate different ways that Americans might decide to restructure the federal government in the face of the strong upward pressure on federal spending coming from an aging population and the rising cost of medical care (table 2-2). Two of these scenarios build on the larger and smaller government

Table 2-2. *Projected Federal Spending, 2030*[a]

Spending as a percent of GDP

Category	Current (2005)[b]	Base-line[c]	Smaller govern-ment[d]	Main-taining the Social Contract[e]	Investing in the Future[f]	Larger govern-ment[g]
Medicare and Medicaid[h]	4.2	11.5	5.7	11.5	8.4	11.5
Social Security[i]	4.2	5.9	5.5	5.9	5.7	5.9
Defense	3.8	2.8	2.0	2.0	2.8	2.8
Other federal spending[j]	6.2	4.3	2.9	2.4	6.1	5.8
Total primary spending	**18.4**	**24.5**	**16.2**	**21.8**	**23.0**	**26.0**
Interest spending[k]	1.5	2.0	2.0	2.0	2.0	2.0
Total spending	**19.8**	**26.5**	**18.2**	**23.7**	**24.9**	**28.0**

Sources: Congressional Budget Office, "The Budget and Economic Outlook: Fiscal Years 2006 to 2015" (January 2005); Congressional Budget Office, "The Long-Term Budget Outlook" (December 2003); Social Security Administration, "Estimates of Financial Effects for Three Models Developed by the President's Commission to Strengthen Social Security" (January 2002); Social Security Administration, "2004 OASDI Trustees Report" (March 2004).

a. Sums may not add to totals because of rounding.

b. Authors' categorization of Congressional Budget Office, "The Budget and Economic Outlook" (January 2005).

c. Scenario 1 from Congressional Budget Office, "The Long-Term Budget Outlook" (December 2003): 2.5 percent excess cost of growth of medical services; Social Security benefits paid as due; defense spending follows FYDP through 2022 and then grows at rate of CPI; nondefense discretionary spending phases down to 3.6 percent of GDP by 2008 (CBO high-spending path).

d. No excess cost of growth of medical services (CBO low-spending path); Social Security benefits indexed to prices; defense spending phases down gradually to $380 billion (2003 dollars) in 2022 and then grows at rate of CPI (CBO low-spending path); a proportional decrease in discretionary spending is added based on *Restoring Fiscal Sanity's* smaller government plan.

e. Two and a half percent excess cost of growth of medical services (CBO high-spending path); Social Security benefits paid as due; defense spending phases down gradually to $380 billion (2003 dollars) in 2022 and then grows at rate of CPI (CBO low-spending path); proportional decrease in discretionary spending is added based on *Restoring Fiscal Sanity's* smaller government plan. Despite the fact that under this plan "other federal spending" is shown to be 0.5 percent less of GDP than under the smaller government plan, both plans have the same amount of money available for programs. The difference occurs because of the different excess cost growth of medical care assumptions under each scenario and their corresponding effects on the Medicare premium offsets accounted for by CBO in the other federal spending category.

f. One percent excess growth of medical cost (CBO intermediate-spending path); Social Security benefits indexed to wages and prices; nondefense discretionary spending phases down to 3.6 percent of GDP by 2008 (CBO high-spending path); 1.5 percent of GDP for additional spending on domestic social programs and international aid.

g. Two and a half percent excess cost of growth of medical services (CBO high-spending path): Social Security benefits paid as due; defense spending follows FYDP through 2022 and then grows at rate of CPI (CBO high-spending path); 1.5 percent of GDP for additional spending on domestic social programs and international aid.

h. As noted in chapters 1 and 4, major uncertainties exist about the future costs of Medicare and Medicaid.

i. The outlays of the price indexing plan were estimated using the SSA memo on the President's Commission to Strengthen Social Security Model 2 as a basis for scaling the change in spending resulting from a pure price indexing plan. The hybrid wage and price indexing plan outlays are assumed to be halfway between pure price indexing and the baseline.

j. This number for "other federal spending" varies depending on the excess cost growth of medical services assumed. This occurs because "other federal spending" includes offsets for Medicare premiums.

k. Interest spending will depend heavily on revenue assumptions over the period. Interest spending in 2030 is approximated by taking the average percentage of GDP interest spending over the next ten years using the adjusted baseline. If deficits are not eliminated over the next decade, interest spending will be larger.

plans developed for the coming decade and illustrate the implications of extending them to 2030. The third scenario, "Investing in the Future," shows the consequences of restraining spending on the elderly in order to maintain programs designed to invest in young people and enhance economic growth. The fourth scenario, "Maintaining the Social Contract," shows the drastic cuts in other programs that would be necessary to fund current promises to seniors while keeping taxes from rising as much as under the larger government plan. Total federal spending in 2005 is expected to be almost 20 percent of GDP. Subtracting out interest on the debt, spending is 18.4 percent of GDP. (Interest payments reflect past decisions about deficit financing combined with the level of interest rates—not current decisions about desired levels of government spending. So looking forward we focus on "primary spending" only.) If current policies are not radically changed, primary spending is projected to rise to about 25 percent of GDP by 2030, as shown in column 2 of the table. This huge increase, equal to 6 percent of GDP, is driven by the increased cost of Medicare and Medicaid. If medical care costs continue to rise at their historical rate of 2.5 percent above the rate of increase of per capita GDP, these two programs alone will rise by more than 7 percent of GDP. Social Security, by contrast, will rise by less than 2 percent of GDP, even if current benefits are continued. Other federal spending, both defense and domestic, will rise in real terms, but it is projected to decline as a share of GDP.

While spending is projected to grow to unprecedented levels, revenues are not scheduled to keep pace. In the post–World War II period, revenues have averaged about 18 percent of GDP.[7] Since 2000, revenues have fallen sharply because of the federal tax cuts enacted over the past four years; they are estimated at 16.8 percent of GDP in 2005. Under the progressive U.S. income tax system, revenues gradually creep up as a share of the economy as higher incomes push people into higher tax brackets—so-called real bracket creep. Revenues also will rise as the retirement population grows and pays taxes on distributions of income from their IRAs or 401(k) plans. But the effects of bracket creep or pension distributions are modest compared with those of widely anticipated legislative actions to extend the tax cuts. Over the next decade and beyond, what happens to revenues will depend critically on whether the Bush administration's tax cuts are allowed to expire as provided in current law or whether they are extended as the administration has proposed. The estimated annual cost by 2015 of extending all expiring tax cuts is $520 billion (including debt service), or 2.6 percent of GDP. If one adds in a further amount for adjusting the alternative minimum tax (AMT), the costs are still higher, and the loss of revenues from both extending the tax cuts and "fixing" the AMT would be $583 billion, or close to 3 percent of GDP.

The bottom line is that even if it is assumed that a number of existing tax provisions—such as lower income tax rates, a higher child tax credit, the elimination of the estate tax, and lower rates on capital gains and dividends—will be allowed to expire, the nation faces a growing gap between spending and revenues over the next few decades. If, as many expect, these provisions are made permanent, the gap becomes a yawning chasm. Without any extension of the aforementioned tax cuts, the primary deficit in 2030 amounts to 4.9 percent of GDP. If the tax cuts are extended, it balloons to 7 percent of GDP.[8]

Smaller Government Scenario

The smaller government scenario assumes that the political process works to hold primary federal spending at approximately its current share of GDP because voters simply refuse to accept higher taxes. Restraining spending will require dramatic departures from current policy, especially in Medicare and Medicaid, and the elimination of many government activities. This scenario depends on the emergence of a strong political consensus that the federal government should not grow faster than the economy, along with a willingness to restructure current programs to restrain their growth.

Advocates of restraining government growth believe that higher taxes would be burdensome to individuals and companies and risk damaging economic growth. They also believe that public spending undermines individual responsibility and initiative and that the private sector spends money more efficiently and effectively than any level of government. Many advocates of restricting federal growth also believe that Washington has usurped functions that would be better performed at the state and local level, where governments arguably are in closer touch with their citizens and know what they want.

In constructing the smaller government scenario, we took the specific cuts suggested for the smaller government plan over the next decade and extended them to 2030 (see column 3 of table 2-2). Relative to the 2030 baseline, this reduced "other federal spending"—everything except defense and the big three entitlement programs—by 1.4 percent of GDP. We achieved another 0.8 percent reduction by not allowing defense spending to grow with the economy. Finally, we placed far more responsibility on individuals to prepare for—and pay the costs of—their own health care and retirement. Initial Social Security benefits were increased to keep up with inflation but not with the projected rise in real wages.[9] As a result, benefits would fall by about 18 percent in 2030 and more steeply thereafter. We also assumed that the political process would set strict limits on the amount of health care expenses subsidized by the government. If health care costs continued to grow more rapidly than the economy, individuals and not government would bear the costs. As a result, seniors, low-income people, and the disabled would find their medical expenses absorbing increasing fractions of their incomes. Chapter 4 suggests some ways in which such limits might be crafted and spells out the likely consequences for beneficiaries.

The medical spending reductions combined with the much smaller Social Security checks envisioned in this plan would hit the elderly hard. In fact, it is difficult to imagine such a scenario being acceptable in a society in which large numbers of senior citizens vote. Yet, even with all of these changes, it is not possible to bring costs in line with revenues unless taxes are allowed to return to at least their historical levels as a share of the economy—that is, about 18 percent.

Still, because of bracket creep, tax revenues would eventually be higher than under our baseline assumptions (see chapter 5), so rates could be cut somewhat if desired. Under this scenario, the federal government would remain roughly as large as it is now despite the elimination of most farm and business subsidies, devolution of major federal functions to the states, cutbacks in many allegedly wasteful or ineffective federal programs, and drastic reductions in now-promised benefits under Social Security, Medicare, and Medicaid. This surprising finding simply reflects the fiscal pressures created by a growing elderly population. Even with no increase in spending per elderly person to accommodate the increased health care costs and higher standards of living that will prevail in the future, the sheer size of the older population means that federal programs will absorb an additional 3 percent of GDP. For that reason, in order to keep taxes at their historical levels, it is necessary to restrict defense and the rest of government spending in ways that currently are politically unthinkable.

Larger Government Scenario

At the other extreme, the larger government scenario assumes that the upward pressure on federal spending over coming decades will induce Americans to accept higher taxes as they call on their government to do more. As they contemplate the choices, Americans may reject reductions in currently promised Social Security benefits. They may also be unable to accept the consequences of shifting the rising costs of medical care from the federal government to individuals. At the same time, they may not want to cut back on other federal services to make room in the budget for the growing retirement programs. Indeed, as incomes rise, citizens may demand more support for education, research, and cultural programs; environmental protection; transportation; and other public goods. Concern about growing divisions in U.S. society also may increase. The distribution of income has become more unequal in recent decades, child poverty rates are much higher than in other industrialized countries, and there is emerging evidence that opportunities to move up the ladder have shrunk for those born into lower-income families.[10] Welfare reform has succeeded in moving many of the poor into jobs, but their incomes remain very low.[11] The public may see government support for low-wage workers (the earned income tax credit, child care, worker training, wage insurance) as necessary to maintain support for a free market economy without European-style labor market regulation, such as high mandatory minimum wages and restrictions on laying off workers.

It may also prove exceedingly difficult to cut other government spending to make room for the retirement programs because many government services are labor intensive and their costs rise as real wages increase. Capital investment and the increased use of technology can improve government efficiency, but there is no way to fully automate bedside nursing, the training of military personnel, preschool education, or managing a national park. In the case of medical care, much greater efficiencies in delivery are certainly possible (see chapter 4), but history does not provide encouragement that cost growth will diminish. Medical advances have created highly effective means of improving health and longevity, but they have generally increased the demand for health care and per capita health care costs.

Increasing global interconnectedness and threats to national security may make it impossible to reduce the share of GDP devoted to defense and international affairs and may even force significant increases. Fighting terrorism and ensuring the safety of the United States and its allies is a clear federal responsibility. It is impossible to predict how threats to American security might evolve over the next several decades or how Americans might respond. An optimistic view would be that current efforts will succeed in reducing terrorist threats to a low level and that no unfriendly superpower or nuclear-armed rogue state will emerge to challenge U.S. hegemony. The United States might then be able to maintain forces sufficient to handle occasional regional threats to the peace around the world and contribute to multilateral peacekeeping, humanitarian, and economic development efforts while maintaining defense and international spending at less than their current share of GDP. A pessimistic view could include continued escalation of militant Islamic terrorist activity; credible nuclear threats from North Korea, Iran, or elsewhere; or the emergence of a hostile government in China intent on military confrontation with the United States. A less frightening, but no less expensive alternative might include the realization that the best hope for American security lies not in more weaponry, but in massive investment designed to raise the standard of living in the poorer parts of Asia, Africa, and Latin America.

The larger government plan spends an additional $420 billion (2004 dollars), as detailed in table 2-3.[12] The plan, which is intended to illustrate what could be accomplished with that level of funding, includes providing a high-quality preschool education for all children under the age of five, with fees based on parental income (estimated cost, $47 billion). It also includes additional federal funding to improve elementary and secondary education. A large portion of those funds would be used to

Table 2-3. *Larger Government Scenario*

Category	Billions of dollars
Higher education[a]	10
K–12 education[b]	40
Pre-K[c]	47
Child care[d]	51
Health care[e]	167
Wage supplements[f]	14
Official development aid[g]	79
Revenue sharing with states	12
Total	420

a. Increases the existing Pell grant program by 75 percent so that, maintaining current eligibility, every grant recipient will get a 75 percent larger grant than under the current system.

b. Primarily devoted to increased funding for teacher quality and training, with about $10 billion left over for other increases in funding for K–12 initiatives. Source: Matthew Miller, *The 2 Percent Solution* (New York: Public Affairs, 2003).

c. Establishes a full-year program with income-related fees and demand-based hours for all children under five years of age. Source: Richard N. Brandon, "Financing Access to Early Education for Children Age Four and Below: Concepts and Costs," paper prepared for the Brookings–University of North Carolina Conference on Creating a National Plan for the Education of Four-Year-Olds," September 9–10, 2004 (revised October 2004).

d. After-school child care for children five to thirteen years of age from families in the bottom four deciles of the income distribution (below about $34,000).

e. Provides federal funding for voluntary, open-access, state-operated insurance pools allowing individuals the option of various privately run health plans at various premium levels. Reduced premiums would be available to low- and middle-income participants. The plan would be open to both employers and individuals and would base its premium on average costs for the non-Medicare population throughout the community. Source: Economic and Social Research Institute, "Covering America: Real Remedies for the Uninsured," June 2001 (www.esresearch.org/covering_america.php [March 17, 2005]).

f. Increase the earned income tax credit so that a full-time, minimum wage worker with two or more children would receive an increase of 14 percent.

g. Implement the recommendations of the UN Millennium Project by devoting 0.7 percent of GNP to official development aid by 2015 and then holding spending constant with inflation and population.

improve the quality of teaching through in-service training and much higher salaries for new teachers combined with reforms that link pay to performance more closely (estimated cost, $40 billion).[13] Access to post-secondary schooling is enhanced by increasing the amount of funding for Pell grants by 75 percent (estimated cost, $10 billion). For an average recipient, the federal grant would increase from about $2,500 a year to more than $4,300. Federal grants to the states for child care are expanded to cover all children under the age of fourteen in families with an income of below four-fifths of median income that are not already covered by other programs (estimated cost, $51 billion). The earnings of low-income working families are given a boost by increasing the earned income tax credit (estimated cost, $14 billion).

By far the most expensive item on this list is health care (estimated cost, $167 billion), which represents the provision of subsidized insurance to low- and moderate-income families through state-run, voluntary insurance pools. Private insurers would compete to provide a basic package of health care services to the non-elderly, thereby improving the efficiency of the system and sharply reducing the number of uninsured Americans.

To reduce human suffering and global poverty while countering the spread of terrorism, the plan provides additional international assistance sufficient to achieve the Millennium Development Goal of 0.7 percent of GNP by 2015 (estimated cost, $79 billion). This goal was set with the objective of halving extreme poverty in developing countries.[14]

Finally, the plan allocates $12 billion for grants to the states based on their population, their wealth, and their own tax-raising efforts. They could then choose whether to spend more on education, highways or mass transit, urban or rural housing or redevelopment, the environment, crime, or other high-priority needs. The advantage of this kind of flexible grant program is that it raises the funds using a broad-based, progressive tax system at the federal level and distributes them to the areas most in need while allowing governors and other state leaders the freedom to set priorities and find more innovative solutions to their problems.

To pay for this plan, people would have to be willing to pay higher taxes. As described in chapter 5, the required revenues could be raised by allowing recent tax cuts to expire, closing loopholes, and creating a new, broad-based consumption tax, such as a 10 percent value-added tax on most expenditures.

A big drawback of this scenario is its cost. Revenues as a share of GDP in 2030 would be about 10 percentage points higher than under the smaller government scenario. The needed revenues could be raised as described in table 5-1 of chapter 5. To put these additional revenues in context, it should be noted that other industrialized countries currently live with much higher taxes than the United States. For example, in 2005 total taxes collected in each of seventeen countries—including the United Kingdom, Germany, the Netherlands, Belgium, and France—will amount to at least 10 percent more of GDP in those countries than do total taxes in the United States.[15] (Including all taxes collected at the local, state, and federal level, the ratio of taxes to GDP is 31 percent in the United States.)

It also is worth noting that with continued growth in the economy, incomes will be much higher in 2030 than they are now. Specifically, real average household income will grow from $67,000 a year in 2005 to about $96,000 in 2030. So even though taxes will take a bigger bite out of people's incomes, because their incomes will be so much higher, after-tax incomes will still increase by 25 percent under the larger government scenario.[16] The issue is not whether this level of government is affordable; it is whether citizens want to devote some of their additional income to the kinds of public uses outlined in this scenario.

Maintaining the Social Contract

This scenario maintains the social contract with senior citizens by down-sizing the rest of government. The emphasis is on keeping existing commitments to the elderly by continuing to provide the benefits currently promised under Social Security, Medicare (including prescription drug coverage), and Medicaid. But to do so without a very large increase in tax rates requires major cutbacks in defense and domestic spending programs. Indeed, the rest of government would need to have its funding cut to the bone.[17] By 2030, domestic spending outside of homeland security would be at its lowest level since data were first collected in 1960. That would mean far fewer resources for the environment, public safety, research, education, housing, unemployment insurance, child care, school lunches, farm subsidies, clean water, law enforcement, and most other such needs.

Although it is unlikely that such a scenario would ever come to pass, it illustrates the enormous fiscal pressures associated with the rising costs of health care and retirement—what some have called "the big squeeze."[18] Because they are entitlements, these health care and retirement programs are now on automatic pilot, whereas most of the programs that serve younger families and their children are vulnerable to cutbacks during the annual appropriations process in Congress. Moreover, because of the political clout of the elderly, it is harder to constrain spending on the health and retirement benefits that they receive. In one manifestation of that clout, one regularly hears elected officials, including the president, say that they will not cut benefits for those who have already retired or are about to retire. No such commitment is made to working-age families that rely on various government benefits, from child care subsidies to health care, even though they often have far fewer resources to fall back on than many of the elderly.

Investing in the Future

This scenario is the mirror image of the plan to maintain the social contract. It curbs spending on the elderly, although not nearly as much as in the smaller government scenario, but it invests more generously in the future-oriented programs and policies, as does the larger government plan. In the end, it imposes a lower tax bill than does the plan to maintain the social contract, and if one believes that future-oriented investments have longer-term payoffs for the economy, then it might cost even less. For example, if investments in education and in better functioning transportation systems lead to more productive workers with higher incomes, those investments would produce higher revenues at any given set of tax rates. The key to making this scenario a reality lies in finding ways to control the growth of health care costs (in our scenarios, from 2.5 percent "excess medical cost inflation" to 1.0 percent). Doing so could involve some combination of guaranteeing a controlled level of subsidy for health care insurance ("premium support"), providing catastrophic coverage only, or rationing care based on more evidence about its effectiveness (see chapter 4). Beyond that, some savings can be gleaned by indexing initial Social Security benefits so that they continue to rise in real terms but not as rapidly as real wages. That approach would put a floor under retirement incomes but place greater responsibility on individuals to save during their working years. However, the budgetary savings from these changes in Social Security benefits pale in comparison to what can be achieved through lower health care costs.

Conclusion

The task of balancing the budget over the next decade is formidable. As illustrated in this chapter, it would take deep spending cuts or substantial new revenues. A more rapid rate of economic growth than currently anticipated or a much slower rate of increase in health care costs could ease the task, but counting on such fortuitous developments would not be wise. Indeed, the next decade will mark only the beginning of what promises to be an unprecedented challenge: how to balance the budget over the longer term as the population ages. To achieve that goal will require Americans either to pay higher taxes than in the past (at least another 6 percent of GDP) or to sharply reduce current levels of support for the elderly by asking them to pay far more for their own health care and retirement. A third alternative—which is to squeeze down most other government programs—will prove inadequate to the task and detrimental to the well-being of younger families and children.

For those who believe that taxes are already too high and government too large and intrusive, we have illustrated the kinds of specific cuts in both entitlements and the rest of government spending that will be required to both balance the budget over the next decade and prevent it from expanding as the population ages. The startling reality here is that even draconian cutbacks in promised benefits to the elderly are insufficient to offset the fiscal pressures created by the sheer increase in their numbers.

For those who find this path of deep spending cuts distasteful, we have crafted a scenario that requires paying substantially higher taxes (an additional 8 percent of GDP, compared with the historical average). That scenario would move the United States closer to accepting the tax levels that prevail in most other industrialized countries but permit greater investment in a range of priorities including education, health care, and assistance to poorer countries and local communities here at home.

Notes

1. The federal government also pursues various objectives through the tax system. For more discussion of these "tax expenditures," see chapter 5.

2. Spending cuts were calculated by assuming an equal reduction in total spending each year between 2004 and 2015 so that the deficit would be eliminated by 2015. About 75 percent of the spending cuts came from discretionary programs; the remainder of the reduction in spending is due to lower interest costs.

3. If we had excluded surpluses in Social Security and Medicare from the budget, we would have set ourselves a deficit reduction target of $1 trillion, but the lower target seemed difficult enough.

4. For a related effort, see Chris Edwards, "Downsizing the Federal Government," Policy Analysis 515 (Washington: Cato Institute, June 2, 2004). Edwards argues that federal spending can be reduced to 17.6 percent of GDP by 2009 by terminating some programs, devolving responsibilities to state or local governments, and privatizing other functions. He cuts a total of $300 billion in FY2004 outlays.

5. These deficit figures are adjusted to extend expiring tax provisions, to adjust the AMT, and to keep discretionary spending per capita constant. Defense spending includes supplementary spending on Iraq, Afghanistan, the global war on terror, and domestic military operations for homeland security.

6. Spending as a proportion of GDP has averaged 20 percent for the past fifty years. Congressional Budget Office, "The Long-Term Budget Outlook" (December 2003), p. 2.

7. Congressional Budget Office, "The Budget and Economic Outlook" (January 2005), figure 4-1.

8. While the effects of interest costs are difficult to predict exactly, it is safe to say that adding interest into the mix will exacerbate the problem.

9. In computing initial benefits, earnings in past years are increased by the amount that average real wages have risen since the wages were earned. After retirement, benefits are indexed to consumer price changes.

10. Gary Burtless and Christopher Jencks, "American Inequality and Its Consequences," in Agenda for the Nation, edited by Henry J. Aaron, James M. Lindsay, and Pietro S. Nivola (Brookings, 2003), pp. 61–108.

11. Isabel V. Sawhill and others, Welfare Reform and Beyond: The Future of the Safety Net (Brookings, 2002).

12. This represents an extra 1.5 percent of GDP in 2030, together with a "growth dividend" (the additional dollars yielded from keeping constant the ratio of "other federal spending" to GDP).

13. Matthew Miller, The 2 Percent Solution (New York: Public Affairs, 2003), p. 126.

14. UN Millennium Project, Investing in Development: A Practical Plan to Achieve the Millennium Development Goals (New York: United Nations Development Program, 2005).

15. Organization for Economic Cooperation and Development, Economic Outlook 76 Database, Annex table 26 (www.oecd.org/dataoecd/5/51/2483816.xls [March 14, 2005]).

16. At 18 percent of GDP, taxes are roughly $14,000 per household (.18 × 1.2 × $67,000). By 2030, under the larger government plan, taxes would need to be about $30,000 (.26 × 1.2 × $96,000). The 1.2 multiplier is the estimated ratio of GDP to personal income.

17. Despite the fact that under this plan "other federal spending" is shown to be 0.5 percent less of GDP than under the smaller government plan, both plans

have the same amount of money available for programs. The difference occurs because of the different excess cost growth of medical care assumptions under each scenario and their corresponding effects on the Medicare premium offsets accounted for by CBO in the other federal spending category.

18. C. Eugene Steuerle, "The Incredible Shrinking Budget for Working Families and Children," National Budget Issues Policy Brief 1 (Washington: Urban Institute, 2003).

3

Social Security

PETER R. ORSZAG AND
JOHN B. SHOVEN

ocial Security plays an important role in the lives of senior citizens. Social Security benefits represent an important source of income for most recipients, and an essential one for some; benefits account for more than half of total income for about two-thirds of beneficiaries over age sixty-five. At the end of December 2004, the average monthly benefit for retired workers was $955, and the average for retired couples was $1,574. Social Security also affects the nation's finances. On the revenue side, Social Security will collect about $600 billion in payroll tax revenue in 2005, accounting for more than a quarter of all federal revenue. For 63 percent of families, Social Security payroll tax exceeds income tax liability.[1] On the expenditure side, Social Security's payments this year will exceed $500 billion, which represents more than a fifth of all Federal outlays.

The primary reason that both Presidents Clinton and George W. Bush have made reforming Social Security a priority is that the system faces a long-term deficit.[2] Under current law, its benefit payments are projected to exceed payroll tax revenue beginning in 2018, and to exceed total revenue (including interest paid to Social Security by the rest of the budget) in 2028. If nothing were done, those deficits would become increasingly large over time. The deficits reflect many factors, including ongoing improvements in life expectancy and the low fertility rates of the past forty years (which are projected to persist in the future). Over the next seventy-five years, the actuarial deficit in the program amounts to 0.7 percent of gross domestic product; over an infinite horizon, the actuarial deficit amounts to 1.2 percent of GDP.

Restoring the solvency of Social Security necessarily involves politically painful choices: either revenue increases or benefit reductions, or some combination of both. Unfortunately, too many analysts and politicians have responded to these unpleasant alternatives by desperately trying to avoid them: they either ignore the need to reform the program or embrace "free lunch" approaches that pretend the problem can be addressed through magic asterisks or gimmicks. The public may be confused by such denials of the problem. A recent poll found that about half of Americans favored leaving Social Security "as is."[3] Regrettably for them, "as is" is not an option over the long run. Avoiding real reform either through delay or by adopting a free lunch approach merely exacerbates the painful choices that will ultimately be necessary to restore solvency and honor whatever benefits have been promised.

As the authors of this chapter, we do not agree on several important issues relating to Social Security. For example, we differ on what would be the appropriate mix of tax increases and benefit reductions to restore long-term balance to the program and on whether some payroll tax revenue should be used for individual accounts. We also disagree about the extent to which the Social Security trust fund has raised national saving and therefore represents real wealth available to help future generations. Despite our differences, we agree on many fundamental issues. We agree that it would be better to eliminate the projected solvency problem sooner rather than later, and that reforms should aim to raise national saving and fairly distribute the necessary burden of eliminating the long-term deficit. Perhaps most important, we both firmly reject the false claims of painless solutions to the projected imbalance in Social Security.

Given these areas of agreement and disagreement, the rest of this chapter is organized into three sections. In the next section we propose objectives for reform of the program. Then, we examine two controversial issues: the economic significance of the Social Security trust fund and the role of individual accounts in reform. Finally, we present and evaluate a menu of options to enhance revenues or reduce obligations. These include, among other possible steps, raising the age of eligibility for collecting full benefits, changing the way initial benefits are determined, and raising the cap on taxable earnings.

Objectives of Reform

Social Security reform necessarily involves a balancing of many competing objectives. In this section, we lay out several key goals for reforming the program.[4]

Objective 1: Reform sooner rather than later. The earlier reform to Social Security is enacted, the more manageable the required adjustments can be: by beginning sooner, it is possible to spread the costs over a longer period of time and ensure that no generation bears an excessive burden. If reform is delayed, by contrast, more dramatic steps will be necessary— including the likelihood of having to make substantial and sudden changes to benefits upon which people had based their retirement plans.

To get some sense of the importance of acting sooner rather than later, consider for illustrative purposes the magnitude of the benefit reductions required to close the entire seventy-five-year deficit solely by reducing nondisability benefits. If benefits were reduced immediately, the required reduction would be slightly less than 15 percent. If the reductions did not begin until 2042, when the Social Security trust fund is projected to be exhausted under current law, the required reduction would be about 30 percent.[5]

These figures actually *understate* the growing problem created by delay, because they assume that all nondisability benefits are reduced— including those for people who have already retired. Substantial benefit reductions for those who are already retired or about to retire, however, are socially undesirable and politically unlikely. President Bush has announced that benefits for those older than fifty-five would not be altered in any plan that had his support. All serious proposals include such protection. However, this feature, while sensible, means larger benefit reductions for everyone else.[6]

Objective 2: Eliminate the Social Security deficit without gimmicks or magic asterisks. Reform should not only eliminate the seventy-five-year deficit in Social Security, but also ensure that another seventy-five-year deficit is not likely to appear in the near future.[7] The problem shouldn't simply be pushed into year seventy-six and beyond. Nor should the deficit be eliminated through other gimmicks or magic asterisks. For example, the budget outside Social Security is projected to be in massive deficit as the baby boomers retire and real health care costs continue to rise. In this context, claiming to eliminate the deficit in Social Security with substantial, unspecified transfers from general revenue amounts to a massive "magic asterisk."

Many reform plans also count the higher expected rate of return on stocks relative to bonds as a deficit-reducing measure. Yet most, if not all, of the higher expected return on stocks reflects risk, and failure to adjust for that risk presents a misleading picture of the budgetary and economic impact of stock investments. Plans that simply assume that the higher expected return on stocks will generate resources to close the deficit and ignore the additional risks associated with stocks are deceptive.

Objective 3: Raise national saving. The issue of how generous a Social Security system the nation can afford in the future depends in part on the nation's ability to produce more goods and services in the future. A Social Security burden that appears onerous under one projection of future national income will be less so if national income grows more rapidly. The future size of the economy depends on many factors, but one of the most important is how much Americans save and invest. Higher national saving increases the size of the capital stock owned by Americans, and increases future national income.

There are many ways in which the federal government can increase national saving, and Social Security is just one of these. But one of the stated motivations for eliminating the long-term deficit in Social Security is to raise national saving. This motivation underscores the shortcomings in plans that assume massive transfers from the rest of the budget (more borrowing) or fail to either reduce benefits or increase revenue. Such plans often generate little or no increase in national saving.

Objective 4: Maintain an adequate replacement rate in the form of an inflation-protected lifetime annuity. Social Security exists in large part because of a concern that workers would not otherwise adequately prepare for retirement on their own. Furthermore, benefits are provided in the form of an inflation-protected lifetime annuity, so that individuals do not face the risk of having their benefit levels eroded by inflation or the risk of outliving their assets. Although some changes to the program are necessary, reform should recognize the fact that myopia and imperfect decisionmaking are not going to disappear. For this and other reasons, including the well-being of the elderly, we should not dramatically reduce the replacement rate from Social Security—that is, the share of a worker's previous earnings that Social Security benefits replace.

Objective 5: Protect the most vulnerable. Social Security has many features that provide relatively larger benefits to the groups with the greatest needs. These groups include surviving spouses, young surviving children, people who have had long careers at low wages, and disabled workers. Social Security reform should include protections for these groups, but they should be targeted as efficiently as possible to relieve hardship at the least cost.

Trust Funds and Individual Accounts

Two key elements of the current Social Security debate are the significance of the Social Security trust fund and the desirability of individual accounts. It is possible to disagree on both of these issues, as the two of us do, for the reasons described in this section.

The Nature of the Social Security Trust Fund

Social Security has been running a cash-flow surplus for the past twenty years and is expected to continue to do so for at least another thirteen years. In short, the system has been collecting more payroll taxes than are necessary to pay current benefits. The excess cash has been turned over to the rest of the government in return for special-issue U.S. government bonds. These bonds earn interest, which is paid by the rest of the government by crediting the Social Security trust fund with more bonds. At the end of 2004, the trust fund stood at about $1.7 trillion. No one should doubt the value of these assets; they are backed by the full faith and credit of the U.S. government. They represent the surpluses of the system—the present value of the extra revenue collected compared to expenditures—over the past twenty years.

Economists debate, however, whether Social Security's surpluses and its trust fund represent an accumulation of wealth that will help future generations in any way. The question is, What happened to the payroll tax money once it was handed over to the rest of the government? Was it saved or spent? Some economists have found that the Social Security surpluses allowed the rest of the government to spend more and tax less than it otherwise would have, implying that the Social Security surpluses had no net effect on the overall unified deficit or national saving.[8] Other economists have reached a different conclusion. They believe that a substantial fraction of the Social Security surplus was used to lower the publicly held debt of the government, thus contributing to national saving.[9]

This difference in view affects one's interpretation of the relative importance of some key dates related to Social Security's finances. The intermediate cost projection from the Social Security trustees suggests that the cash-flow Social Security surplus (that is, the surplus excluding interest paid from the rest of the government to Social Security) will continue to increase as a share of payroll until 2007. The cash-flow surplus then begins to decline rather dramatically as the baby boomers begin to collect retirement benefits in significant numbers. By around 2018, the cash-flow surplus will disappear. However, payroll taxes and interest earned on trust fund bonds will cover all benefits until 2028. At that point, the system will have to begin to sell its stock of special-issue bonds back to the rest of the government. These sales will continue until the bonds are exhausted, in roughly 2042.

Those who believe the trust fund has raised national saving tend to focus on the 2042 date, since the additional saving they believe it has produced will better prepare the nation for the claim on general revenues entailed by interest and principal payments on the trust fund bonds between 2018 and 2042. Those who do not believe that the trust fund has improved national saving tend to focus on 2018, since that is the point at which the program's cash flow turns negative and claims on general revenue begin.

Individual Accounts

Social Security has always featured a pay-as-you-go defined benefit retirement system. By *defined benefit* we simply mean that benefits are determined by formula and not by investment returns. Social Security has a different structure, however, from anything in the private sector. In particular, a defined benefit system in the private sector alters the firm's required contributions in response to changes in life expectancy, investment returns, or work patterns. Under Social Security, by contrast, the contributions (in particular the payroll tax), as well as the payments, are legislated and determined by formula. Social Security thus currently lacks the full built-in flexibility of private sector pensions—even those that offer a defined benefit—although the system is also indexed to various factors that reflect economic developments.

The private sector has been moving at a rapid pace from defined benefit plans to defined contribution plans. Social Security reform recommendations with defined contribution elements, or individual accounts, gained prominence during the proceedings of the 1994–96 Advisory Council on Social Security; since then, many proposals have included individual accounts. Interest in such accounts is probably strongest amongst those who believe that Social Security's cash-flow surpluses have failed to increase national saving. Opposition is strongest amongst those who believe that defined contribution plans and their associated risks do not belong in the core tier of retirement income, especially when the private pension system is also shifting toward defined contribution plans.

There are two ways to fund individual accounts, referred to as *add-on* or *carve-out*. Add-on plans would require contributions over and above the payroll tax used to finance traditional retirement benefits under Social Security. Carve-out plans would divert some portion of existing payroll taxes into individual accounts. An important point is that neither carve-out nor add-on plans are free, from the participant's point of view. The payment for the carve-out plans comes when benefits are subsequently reduced to offset the cost of the revenue deposited into the account. Under Model 2 from the President's Commission to Strengthen Social Security, for instance, those who voluntarily participate in the individual accounts program have their regular Social Security checks reduced by an amount that equals (in expected present value) the amount they diverted into the account plus interest (at an interest rate of 2 percentage points plus inflation). With add-on accounts, the cost is more immediate and comes in the form of the extra contributions that the participants make. Any returns from these contributions subsequently add to their retirement income.

A feature of carve-out plans, such as Model 2, is that they create a cash-flow problem. Between the time when revenue is diverted into the accounts and when it is "paid back" through reductions in regular benefits, the program has less money available to pay the benefits of those currently retired. To be sure, the combined effect of the individual accounts and the benefit changes unrelated to the accounts under Model 2 is a surplus within Social Security in 2058 and beyond. But the plan nonetheless raises public debt for about six decades, because the negative cash flow from the accounts dominates the positive effect from the benefit changes for an extended period. Economists hold different views regarding the degree to which the extra borrowing during this transition period would drive up interest rates or pose fiscal risks.

According to their advocates, add-on accounts are the most promising way to increase national saving. This would be particularly true if participation were mandatory rather than voluntary. Some participants in an add-on system, whether mandatory or voluntary, would reduce other forms of saving, so the net addition to private saving would be considerably lower than the total contributions to the plan. It is impossible to predict exactly the extent of such offsetting, but it is likely to be a higher share of contributions under a voluntary system than a mandatory one.

On the issue of risk, we agree with each other and with most other economists that individual accounts invested in publicly traded stocks and bonds would be risky. However, especially in the absence of reform, traditional Social Security benefits also carry risks. Currently promised benefits are underfunded and are likely to be reduced in one way or another. In addition, even an actuarially balanced system could still be affected by uncertainties surrounding future rates of fertility, mortality, immigration, and productivity.

Proponents of individual accounts argue that people can choose how much risk to take. They also like the fact that the balances in such accounts can be bequeathed. Opponents of individual accounts argue that the foundation of retirement income is not the place to take inappropriate risks, and that the accounts could be burdened by high administrative costs. They also note that the defined contribution nature of accounts could create political pressures to allow pre-retirement withdrawals or less than full annuitization upon retirement.

Individual accounts by themselves will not reduce the underlying deficit in Social Security. Either benefit promises under the current system have to be reduced or additional revenues identified. Add-on individual accounts are actuarially fair, by definition: they are self-financing and do not generate any surplus money to help meet existing Social Security promises. Carve-out individual accounts can also be designed to be roughly actuarially fair (as under the Bush administration's proposal in 2005, which slightly modified the proposal from the President's Commission to Strengthen Social Security); such actuarially neutral accounts neither increase nor reduce the projected deficit over an infinite horizon. The only indirect way that individual accounts could help address solvency is by somehow making reducions in traditional Social Security benefits more politically acceptable. An add-on individual account, in particular, would increase the retirement resources of participants and possibly make it more acceptable to reduce traditional Social Security benefits; of course, the add-on accounts also mean that workers must contribute more to their own retirement. If these contributions were mandatory, many observers (likely including the official budget scorers) would call them a tax.

It is worth noting that many opponents of carve-out accounts strongly support individual accounts in the form of 401(k)s and IRAs. That is, they believe that such accounts have a critical role to play in filling the hole between the foundation provided by Social Security and a comfortable retirement. These economists argue that although individual accounts make sense on top of Social Security, they do not make sense as part of the core retirement income provided by the program. Within that core, benefits should continue to be provided in a form that is protected against inflation, does not fluctuate with the stock market, and lasts as long as you are alive.

A Menu of Options

We have tried to state the problem as simply as possible. Over the long run, Social Security does not have enough revenues to meet its promises. The 2004 trustees' report for Social Security estimates that the present value of benefits exceeds the present value of receipts (plus the trust fund) over the next seventy-five years by 1.89 percent of the present value of the payroll tax base ("covered payroll"). They also estimate that the revenue shortfall at the end of the seventy-five-year period, in 2078, will be 5.91 percent of covered payroll. In other words, it would take roughly a 6 percent of payroll increase in revenues or a similar reduction in benefits to achieve solvency in that year. As already noted, we believe the goal should be to achieve financial balance over the next seventy-five years and to avoid the rapid appearance of another seventy-five-year deficit, which requires avoiding significant deficits at the end of the seventy-five-year period. Table 3-1 lists the measures we discuss below and their percentage contribution toward achieving these goals.

Reducing Promised Benefits

There are obviously numerous ways to reduce retirement benefits. We focus on those that take effect gradually, since we think that is both socially and politically desirable.

1. INDEXING INITIAL BENEFITS BY PRICE RATHER THAN WAGE INFLATION. Currently, initial Social Security benefits increase with average wages in the economy.[10] This means that if wages go up more rapidly than prices over the long haul, monthly retirement benefits increase in real terms. Under the intermediate set of assumptions of the Social Security trustees, people retiring in 2050 would get monthly benefits approximately 64 percent higher in real terms than those of today's retirees, since their lifetime wages would be that much higher. This system generates a constant replacement rate (that is, the share of pre-retirement earnings replaced by Social Security) from one generation to the next under Social Security.

In Model 2 of the President's Commission to Strengthen Social Security, initial benefits would instead be linked only to price increases, not

Table 3-1. *Impact of Alternative Reform Measures
on Social Security's Solvency*

Proposal	Percentage improvement in	
	75-year imbalance	75th-year cash-flow deficit
Replace wage indexing with price indexing (president's commission Model 2 without individual accounts)	101	116
Hybrid indexing	71	70
Accelerate increase in full benefit age to 67, index FBA by 1 month every 2 years until FBA = 70	36	29
Increase number of years in benefit calculation from 35 to 40	22	11
Change benefit formula: multiply 22 and 15 percent factors by 0.987 each year, to reduce to 21 and 10 percent in 2035	85	57
Subject 90 percent of earnings to payroll tax and credit them for benefit purposes	40	14
Raise payroll tax rates by 2 percentage points effective in 2005 (employer + employee)	104	34

Source: U.S. Social Security Administration (SSA), Office of Chief Actuary, "Estimates of Financial Effects for Three Models Developed by the President's Commission to Strengthen Social Security," Memorandum, January 31, 2002; SSA, Office of Chief Actuary, "Preliminary Estimates for a Proposal to Reduce Benefits above the Level Provided at the 30th Percentile under Present Law," Memorandum to Bob Pozen from Steve Goss, August 21, 2003; and SSA, Office of Chief Actuary, "Estimated OASDI Long-Range Financial Effects of Several Provisions Requested by the Social Security Advisory Board," Memorandum to Stephen C. Goss, Chief Actuary, from Chris Chaplain, Actuary, Alice H. Wade, Deputy Chief Actuary, February 7, 2005.

wage increases. This amounts to eliminating the real increase in future Social Security benefits (since they would only keep up with prices, not wages) and would cause the replacement rate to decline continuously over time. By 2050, benefits for new retirees would be 39 percent lower than projected under current law, and the average replacement rate would be approximately 25 percent rather than the 43 percent that prevails today.

This shift in the way initial benefits are determined would have a very large effect on Social Security's solvency: The chief actuary of Social Security has estimated that this change alone would more than eliminate the seventy-five-year deficit and result in the system running a surplus beyond the seventy-five-year horizon.[11]

Proponents of price indexing initial benefits argue that it offers a way to restore Social Security's solvency without reducing benefits below the inflation-adjusted level enjoyed by today's retirees. Opponents argue that the replacement rate is a natural way to gauge the adequacy of the safety net provided by Social Security, and the index switch amounts to a gradual but ultimately dramatic diminution of one of the primary social insurance functions of the system.

2. HYBRID INDEXING. Pozen, Schieber, and Shoven have suggested a change in the indexation of initial benefits that preserves the most important safety net features of Social Security.[12] They propose wage indexing the benefits for those with low lifetime earnings and price indexing the benefits for high income participants. Under this approach, those least able to absorb cuts (the bottom 30 percent of the lifetime earnings distribution) are exempt from the benefit reductions.[13]

Gradually, the whole benefit structure would become significantly more progressive, as the replacement rates for higher-income participants were reduced but those for lower-income participants were maintained. Under the Social Security Administration's intermediate cost projections, those with an earnings history in the 30th percentile would receive benefits equal to those with the highest earnings history by around 2090. Eventually, the whole benefit structure would become flat, in that everyone with a full-length career would get the same real monthly benefits.

Hybrid indexing (also known as progressive price indexing) would not reduce overall costs as much as straight price indexing, but it still has a significant effect on Social Security's solvency. In 2003, the chief actuary of Social Security estimated that this hybrid indexing scheme would eliminate approximately 71 percent of Social Security's seventy-five-year deficit. Similarly, it would reduce the shortfall at the end of the seventy-five-year window by 70 percent. Rather than ever-widening deficits in the seventy-sixth year and beyond, hybrid indexing would produce smaller and smaller deficits, and eventually, a surplus.

3. INCREASING THE FULL BENEFIT AGE. The full benefit age (FBA) is the age at which a single individual gets the full monthly benefit determined by the formula linking benefits to prior earnings. Those who retire after sixty-two but before the FBA get less than full benefits, and those who retire later (up to seventy) get more. The FBA is sixty-five for those born before 1983. For those born in 1940, who turned sixty-five in 2005, the FBA is sixty-five years and six months. It is scheduled to increase in

an uneven manner until it reaches sixty-seven for those born in 1960. Under current law, it will then remain at sixty-seven indefinitely. Although benefits are adjusted when people retire earlier or later than the FBA, raising the FBA, or normal retirement age, is equivalent to a cut in monthly benefits, regardless of when someone commences benefits.

The rationale for increasing the FBA is that life expectancy has increased very substantially and will likely continue to do so, and that life expectancy raises costs because benefits are received over a longer period, on average. As a rough approximation, each year's new cohort of sixty-five-year-olds can expect to live about three weeks longer than the previous year's cohort. The question is whether all of that extra life should translate into higher lifetime benefits under Social Security. More to the point, longer life expectancies are an important cause of Social Security's financial problems. Increasing the FBA could reduce, eliminate, or in some cases more than compensate for these costs.

There are a variety of ways to increase the FBA. One possibility would be to accelerate the scheduled increase to sixty-seven so that it applies to those born in 1949 (fifty-six-year-olds in 2005) rather than those born in 1960 (forty-five-year olds in 2005). After that, the FBA would increase very gradually for younger workers until it reaches seventy for those born in 2021. This plan would eliminate about 36 percent of the seventy-five-year deficit and about 29 percent of the cash-flow shortfall in the seventy-fifth year.[14]

An alternative way of indexing the system to life expectancy would be to calculate each year the expected cost of improvements in longevity. The monthly benefit formula could then be adjusted to keep lifetime benefits roughly constant as life expectancy increased, thereby insulating the system from changes in life expectancy. This approach would eliminate about one-quarter of the seventy-five-year deficit.[15]

4. INCREASING THE NUMBER OF YEARS USED TO CALCULATE BENEFITS. Social Security currently counts workers' highest thirty-five years of indexed earnings in determining their retirement benefits. There have been proposals to increase the number of years used in the calculation. For instance, Social Security could use the best forty years of indexed earnings in the computation. Clearly, this would be a benefit cut, in that every worker's average indexed earnings will be lower if they are based on

the best thirty-five years plus five years that were not good enough to enter into the old calculation. The benefit reductions would be concentrated on those whose covered careers were thirty-five years or shorter, since the additional years would be entered as zeros. Social Security estimates that moving to a forty-year calculation would lower the promised benefits enough to eliminate 22 percent of the seventy-five-year deficit and 11 percent of the revenue shortfall at the end of the seventy-five-year window, in 2078.

5. CHANGING THE BENEFIT FORMULA. Another way to reduce benefits is a straightforward revision in the benefit formula. The formula determines the benefits of a single worker at the FBA as a function of his or her average indexed monthly earnings (AIME). Because the formula is progressive, replacing a higher fraction of low-wage than of high-wage earnings, there are two "bend" points: in 2005, one at $627 per month and the other at $3,779 per month.[16] Up to the first bend point, the monthly benefit amount is 90 percent of the AIME. Between the two bend points, an extra $1 of AIME results in an extra 32 cents of monthly benefits, and beyond the second bend point an extra $1 of AIME produces an extra 15 cents in benefits. If, for example, the 90 percent rate were left unchanged, but the 32 and 15 percent rates in the formula were gradually reduced to 21 and 10 percent, respectively, by 2035, the impact on solvency would be considerable. Social Security estimates that this particular revision to the benefit formula would eliminate 85 percent of the seventy-five-year deficit and 57 percent of the deficit in 2078, at the end of the seventy-five-year window.

Increasing Revenues

As noted above, some people believe that higher Social Security taxes would result in more government spending (or substitute for other taxes), rather than increasing saving. Others believe that failure to raise revenue will put excessive pressure on future benefits. But both sides agree that from a fiscal perspective, raising the revenues of the system would help its solvency.

1. INCREASING THE EARNINGS CAP SUBJECT TO SOCIAL SECURITY PAYROLL TAXES. Currently, the payroll tax is imposed on taxable earnings

up to $90,000. This cap excludes about 15 percent of total earnings in the economy. Even though the cap is indexed for wage inflation, the proportion of earnings above the cap has increased, due to the widening dispersion of earnings. If the cutoff were increased so that 90 percent instead of 85 percent of total earnings were subject to tax, the cutoff amount would have to be increased to approximately $150,000. Although the extra taxable earnings would increase future benefits, the change would improve the solvency of the system, since all of the extra earnings would be in the third tier of the benefit formula. Social Security estimates that this policy would solve almost 40 percent of the seventy-five-year deficit, but only 14 percent of the 2078 cash-flow deficit.

2. RAISING THE PAYROLL TAX RATE. Another straightforward way to improve the solvency of Social Security is to raise the Social Security payroll tax rate. Raising the combined employer and employee payroll tax to 14.4 percent (from 12.4 percent) would eliminate the entire seventy-five-year deficit. But it would only reduce the cash-flow deficit in 2078 by about one-third.

What We Would Do

As we have noted, we agree on many issues and disagree on others. Given our menu of options, here are our recommendations for Social Security reform:

Orszag would achieve sustainable solvency with a combination of benefit reductions and tax increases. Low-income participants and other vulnerable beneficiaries would be protected from most or all of the benefit cuts. Some of the benefit cuts and tax increases would be indexed to improvements in life expectancy. A complete and detailed plan along these lines is presented in his book with Peter Diamond, *Saving Social Security: A Balanced Approach.*[17]

Shoven, taking into account political feasibility as well as economic attractiveness, would institute hybrid indexing and also index the full benefit age to changes in life expectancy that occur after 2022. Individual accounts could be considered separately, once long-run solvency is restored with these two measures. Shoven would also support more radical reform involving sizable and mandatory individual accounts along with flat traditional Social Security benefits that are more progressive than at present, providing the same basic benefits to all workers. Such a plan is laid out in his book with Sylvester Scheiber, *The Real Deal: The History and Future of Social Security*.[18]

Conclusion

We have tried to emphasize two things over everything else. First, restoring solvency to Social Security requires either increasing contributions to the system or reducing the promised benefits, or some of each. Nothing else will work. Second, taking the necessary steps sooner rather than later has dramatic advantages. We even agree on most of the other goals of Social Security reform. Restoring Social Security's solvency is manageable, particularly if it is done promptly. There are several ways to accomplish the task and make Social Security secure for generations to come. We want to preserve and enhance the progressivity of the system and protect the most vulnerable. Similarly, we both feel that the United States should increase its national saving rate, and that Social Security should be reformed in a way consistent with that goal. We also agree that whatever form Social Security reform takes, many households need to increase their retirement saving over and above what the program provides; recent empirical studies have pointed the way toward accomplishing that goal.[19]

Notes

1. Authors' calculation using Urban-Brookings Tax Policy Microsimulation Model (version 0304-3).

2. Solvency data can be found in U.S. Social Security Administration, "The 2004 Annual Report of the Board of Trustees of the Federal Old-Age and Survivors Insurance and Disability Insurance Trust Funds" (Washington: letter of transmittal dated March 23, 2004).

3. Wall Street Journal/NBC News poll, February 10–14, 2005; reported in Jackie Calmes and John Harwood, "Greenspan Supports Bush on 'Private Accounts': Endorsement Comes as Poll Shows Rising Public Doubt on Social Security Change," *Wall Street Journal*, February 17, 2005, p. A1.

4. Edward Gramlich has also proposed sensible rules for assessing Social Security reform. See Gramlich, "Rules for Assessing Social Security Reform," remarks

at the annual conference of the Retirement Research Consortium, National Press Club, Washington, August 12, 2004.

5. Authors' calculations using benefit data provided by the Social Security Administration.

6. For example, if benefits were reduced this year but only for those aged fifty-four or younger, the required benefit reduction would be about 25 percent. If reform were delayed until 2042 and benefits were reduced only at that time for those fifty-four or younger, the benefit reduction required to achieve seventy-five-year balance would be somewhere between 70 and 90 percent (authors' calculations). In other words, delaying reform means that it becomes increasingly untenable to protect those who are retired or near retirement.

7. Merely eliminating the deficit over the next seventy-five years, while preserving the current structure of Social Security, would result in the appearance of another seventy-five-year deficit as the projection window rolls forward in time. This phenomenon is referred to as the terminal-year problem. For example, the seventy-five-year window for the 2005 projections extends from 2005 through 2079. For the 2006 projection, the actual outcome in 2005 will be included in the initial trust fund balance, and the seventy-five-year window for the projection will shift to 2006 through 2080. Since retirees in the future are expected to live longer, and the system is still transitioning to the effects of lower fertility and immigration rates (resulting in slower growth of the labor force), the program is projected to have a negative net cash flow in 2080. Thus the effect of adding 2080 is to increase the seventy-five-year actuarial imbalance. In our view, reform should ensure that the mere passage of time does not necessarily reintroduce a seventy-five-year deficit.

8. See, for example, Kent Smetters, "Is the Social Security Trust Fund a Source of Value?" *American Economic Review* 94, no. 2, *Papers and Proceedings* (May 2004): 176–81; and Sita Nataraj and John B. Shoven, "Has the Unified Budget Undermined the Federal Government Trust Funds?" paper presented at the annual conference of the Retirement Research Consortium, National Press Club, Washington, August 12–13, 2004.

9. Peter Diamond and Peter Orszag, *Saving Social Security: A Balanced Approach* (Brookings, 2004).

10. After one starts receiving Social Security retirement checks, the monthly benefits are increased annually to keep pace with price inflation (the Consumer Price Index).

11. The Office of the Chief Actuary finds that excluding the individual accounts, Model 2 would roughly eliminate the seventy-five-year imbalance and also result in the program running a surplus at the end of the seventy-five-year window. The index switch alone has bigger effects, because Model 2 involves higher benefits for widows and the lifetime poor that partially offset the indexing effects.

12. Robert Pozen, Sylvester J. Schieber, and John B. Shoven, "Improving Social Security's Progressivity and Solvency with Hybrid Indexing," *American Economic Review* 94, no. 2, *Papers and Proceedings* (May 2004): 187–91.

13. Under their proposal, Social Security would calculate the 30th percentile of the average indexed monthly earnings distribution in 2012. That amount is

projected to be slightly over $2,000 per month. The figure would be indexed after 2012 by the average wage rate in the economy. Anyone whose average indexed lifetime earnings are below this figure (that is, in the bottom 30 percent of retirees in terms of lifetime earnings) would continue to enjoy wage indexed benefits; that is, they would have precisely the same future benefits as currently promised in the law. At the same time, those at the top of the distribution (those whose average indexed earnings are at or above the payroll tax cutoff ($7,500 a month or $90,000 per year in 2005) would have their initial retirement benefits linked to the consumer price index). Those between the 30th percentile and the earnings cap would have their benefits go up faster than prices but slower than wages. Those just above the 30th percentile would have their benefits mostly linked to wages, while those just below the cap would be mostly tied to prices.

14. The full benefit age in 2080 would be approximately 69.5 years.

15. U.S. Social Security Administration, Office of Chief Actuary, "Estimate of Financial Effects for a Proposal to Restore Solvency to the Social Security Program," Memorandum to Peter Diamond, Professor, MIT, Peter Orszag, Senior Fellow, Brookings Institution, from Stephen C. Goss, Chief Actuary, October 8, 2003, p. 2.

16. The bend points increase each year, according to the average wage rate in the economy.

17. Diamond and Orszag, *Saving Social Security*.

18. Sylvester J. Schieber and John B. Shoven, *The Real Deal: The History and Future of Social Security* (Yale University Press, 1999).

19. William G. Gale, J. Mark Iwry, and Peter R. Orszag, "The Automatic 401(k): A Simple Way to Strengthen Retirement Saving," *Tax Notes*, March 7, 2005, pp. 1207–14. See also the Retirement Security Project (www.retirement securityproject.org).

4

Health

HENRY J. AARON AND
JACK MEYER

Projected increases in federal spending on health care programs account for most of the anticipated gap between taxes and spending over the next few decades. The gap is so large that cuts in other government programs cannot plausibly close it. The remaining alternatives are to cut Medicare and Medicaid benefits sharply or to accept huge tax increases. Efforts to eliminate waste and improve efficiency should be pursued and may yield sizable savings, but the savings will not be enough to avoid difficult choices. The problem is just too large, and transforming existing medical practices will take many years.

That challenge is hard enough, but it is only part of the problem. The same hospitals and physicians that care for Medicare and Medicaid patients also serve the privately insured. For decades per capita spending in the private sector has risen at a rate similar to that of the public sector. To seek significantly different standards of care for the populations in the two sectors is neither practicable nor desirable. To significantly lower Medicare and Medicaid costs, it may be necessary to limit care for everyone. In plain terms, closing the federal fiscal gap will likely require health care rationing for all.

The Problem: Rising Health Care Costs

Growth of health care spending has outpaced the increase in income per person for the past half-century by an average of more than 2.5 percentage points a year. The source of most of this increase has been the steady march of medical science, which has generated impressive advances in human well-being. From early antibiotics that quickly cured previously intractable and often lethal infections, to artificial hips and knees and imaging devices that have largely replaced exploratory surgery, these advances have brought enormous benefits.[1]

But the advances have not been cheap. For decades health care spending has claimed ever larger shares of national income, rising from 5.7 percent of gross domestic product in 1965, the year Medicare and Medicaid were enacted, to 15.3 percent in 2003. Federal government expenditures on health, which were a tiny 0.4 percent of gross domestic product in 1965, rose to 4.9 percent in 2004. Well-insured Americans have every reason to seek essentially all beneficial services, however small the benefit and however high the cost. Providers who are paid for each service rendered have every incentive to supply those services. As a result, per capita health spending in the United States exceeds that in every other nation by at least 47 percent.[2]

Nor is the growth in health care spending likely to slow down. Advances in molecular medicine and genomics, along with the aging of the population, promise to turn the stream of innovative diagnostic and therapeutic procedures into a torrent.[3] Rapid increases in the proportion of the population that is aged or disabled, together with government programs that largely serve these groups, mean that growth in federal health care spending will accelerate.

A continuation of past trends, with health care spending growing 2.5 percent a year more than income, may seem relatively benign. Were the differential to persist, however, *federal* spending on health care by 2045 would claim as large a share of national income as the total federal budget (other than interest on the national debt) does today. By 2022, annual increases in total health care spending would absorb more than half of economic growth—and by 2051, all of it.

Table 4-1 shows federal outlays on Medicare and Medicaid as a share of gross domestic product and of federal spending under two alternative

Table 4-1. *Projection of Medicare and Medicaid Expenditures as a Percent of Federal Outlays and of GDP*

| | Medicare and Medicaid outlays | | | |
| | Percent of federal outlays[a] | | Percent of GDP[b] | |
Year	Historical trend scenario[c]	Slowed growth scenario[d]	Historical trend scenario	Slowed growth scenario
2005	19.6	19.6	4.2	4.2
2010	23.2	22.5	5.3	4.8
2020	28.9	27.7	7.8	6.5
2030	33.6	30.8	11.5	8.4
2040	36.1	32.2	16.1	10.1

Source: Figures for 2005 are estimates taken from CBO, "The Budget and Economic Outlook: Fiscal Years 2006 to 2015 (Washington, January 2005). Figures for subsequent years are projections from CBO, "The Long-Term Budget Outlook" (December 2003) (www.cbo.gov/showdoc.cfm?index=4916&sequence=0 [March 17, 2005]).

a. Federal outlays net out premium payments because they are not a share of federal costs. GDP shares are based on the gross cost of services paid in full or in part by Medicare and Medicaid.

b. National outlays on Medicaid as a share of GDP include spending by state and local governments, set at two-thirds of federal outlays.

c. The historical trend scenario assumes that Medicare and Medicaid cost growth exceeds GDP by 2.5 percent a year.

d. The slowed growth scenario assumes that Medicare and Medicaid cost growth exceeds GDP by 1 percent a year.

assumptions—that per capita Medicare and Medicaid outlays continue to increase at the trend rate of 2.5 percentage points a year more than per capita income or that excess spending falls to 1 percentage point a year.

Such projections should provoke two reactions. The first is that mindless extrapolations are, well, *mindless*. Nothing, not even health care costs, can continuously grow materially faster than something of which it is a part. At some point, growth of health care spending must diminish.

The second reaction should be to wonder just *how* the growth of health care spending will be slowed. Were advances in medical science to lower costs rather than boost them, the adjustment would be quite painless. Such an outcome is, however, quite improbable. Scientific advancement often lowers *prices*, but it seldom lowers *cost,* which is price multiplied by quantity.[4] Most important, the trends portrayed in table 4-1 portend some very difficult budgetary choices.

One option is to adopt diverse measures to slow the growth of health care spending in ways that do not undercut the access of the poor, elderly, and disabled to beneficial care or treat them and privately insured Americans differently. The savings from the measures we describe could be significant, although probably not as large as their advocates claim. In particular, they are unlikely to forestall very rapid growth in the share of federal spending devoted to health programs.

If these measures do not control health care spending, the nation will face a nasty dilemma. It could raise taxes sharply—and spend relentlessly increasing shares of private income on health care as well. It could deny beneficial care to some patients—that is, ration care. Or it could require patients to pay directly for a larger share of the cost of care. For reasons described below, we anticipate that the nation is likely to have to do some of all three.

Measures to Curtail the Growth of Health Care Spending

Numerous studies document that the U.S. health care system generates a great deal of care that promises no medical benefit and a distressing amount that is downright harmful.[5] Inappropriate care is not unique to the United States, but certain features of the U.S. health care system may encourage it.[6] The payment system rewards providers for doing more. The threat of litigation frightens them into doing more. Physicians usually practice as they were taught, even if current research does not validate their methods. Poor organization of hospitals and doctor's offices and missed opportunities to use information technology to reduce medical errors cause needless illness and death, although the number of such adverse outcomes often is exaggerated.[7] And, of course, mortals—even physicians—sometimes err.

Such waste and inefficiency can be reduced. Increased use of computers to control the dispensing of medication and to maintain patient records would reduce medical error. Reeducation of physicians and other providers can hasten the introduction of "best practices." Well-designed tort reform may reduce "defensive medicine"—care provided because it protects doctors against litigation, not because it is medically indicated.[8]

A review of forty-eight articles from leading professional journals found that 20 percent of patients received unnecessary or "contraindicated" chronic care and 30 percent received contraindicated acute care. But the same authors also found that 30 percent of patients studied did not receive recommended acute care, 40 percent did not receive recommended chronic care, and 50 percent did not receive recommended preventive care.[9] Furthermore, an Institute of Medicine study found that overuse of services is more likely to be detected than underuse because noticing error in medical records is easier than pinpointing where more should have been done. Those who allege that health care costs could be controlled by eliminating waste are more punctilious in citing statistics on overuse than on underuse.[10] Malpractice reforms that do no more than cap damages may reduce somewhat the incentive to overprovide care created by the threat of unlimited damages and thereby save money. However, they may also lead some providers to offer less care than they should and thereby reduce needed care.

These studies clearly document that medical care is misdirected. They do not show, however, that a system that targets recipients more accurately would cost much less than the existing one. Recent research indicates that Medicare expenditures could be reduced nearly 29 percent without affecting health outcomes if the level of spending in high-cost regions could be reduced to the level in low-cost regions.[11] Such findings hold the tantalizing promise of major savings. But persuading physicians and hospitals in higher-cost cities such as New York and Miami to practice medicine the way it is done in lower-cost cities such as Minneapolis and Seattle is not easy and may take many years to accomplish.

The first message from all of this research is that enacting and implementing measures that simultaneously curtail waste and ensure provision of needed care will take time and money. The second lesson is that precisely because solving these problems will take time, investments should begin promptly. Research on cost-effective medicine is in its infancy. Physicians' habits in practicing medicine are notoriously hard to change. But the possibility of training and mentoring new generations of physicians to keep them up to date at relatively low cost is increasing with computer-based data systems. Such systems also can be used to maintain medical records, order medications and tests, and process patient bills, although they will require the resolution of many as-yet-unsolved problems and large up-front investments.[12]

Inefficiencies and inappropriate care could be reduced by revising payment incentives and by reorganizing the delivery of care into competing integrated delivery networks with limited provider panels. Capping the exclusion from taxes of employer-financed insurance at a level that would cover standard physician and hospital services would encourage businesses and individuals to shop for tightly managed health plans. Consumers would be given incentives not to enroll in high-cost plans, and providers would be rewarded for adhering to best medical practices rather than for providing all possible services. Yet capping the exclusion from personal income and payroll taxes of employer-financed health insurance and fostering plans with tightly limited rosters of health care providers have so far generated little political support.

The Medicare Modernization Act of 2003 contained a provision with some promise for reducing the level of health care spending. Under that provision, people who purchase so-called high-deductible health insurance may deposit sums in highly tax-favored vehicles called health savings accounts (HSAs) that may be used for health expenses at any time during their lives or bequeathed to their heirs for health outlays. The deductibles must be at least $1,000 for individuals and $2,000 for families. Annual deposits in the accounts may not exceed the deductible or a cap.[13] HSAs have some promise of slowing, at least temporarily, the growth of health care spending. They also carry a threat. If they shift healthier-than-average people from group to individual insurance plans, they could raise the average price of traditional group insurance. If they lead to the demise of group insurance, they would force older people and those with chronic illnesses into the individual insurance market, where they would face very high premiums.

Medicare and Medicaid Reforms

Certain changes in Medicare and Medicaid could reduce federal budget outlays. Some would cut total spending. Others would simply shift government spending to private payers.

Raising the Age of Eligibility for Medicare

In 1965, Medicare legislation set the eligibility age at sixty-five, a seemingly natural choice because "full" Social Security benefits were paid at

Table 4-2. *Impact on Medicare Costs of Increasing Medicare Age of Eligibility*[a]

Increased age of eligibility	Savings as a percent of outlays
66	3.0
67	5.8
68	8.8
69	11.9
70	15.1
71	18.6
72	22.3

Source: Authors' calculations based on data from the Congressional Budget Office.

a. The projections are based on data on relative Medicare spending by age of beneficiary for the year 1999, supplied by Tom Bradley of the Congressional Budget Office. We assume that the ratio of expenditures at each age to average Medicare outlays per person persists into the future, as does the proportion of Medicare beneficiaries at each age. Relative expenditures do not include any allowance for added outlays under the Medicare drug benefit added by the Medicare Modernization Act of 2003. In fact, the age composition of the elderly in 2030 will differ little from that in 2005. Whether relative outlays by age will change will depend on the pattern of technological change and payment policy under Medicare.

age sixty-five.[14] Two important developments have occurred since then. First, workers have begun to claim Social Security benefits at progressively earlier ages—more than 70 percent of workers now claim benefits between the ages of sixty-two and sixty-five. This shift might imply lowering the age of eligibility for Medicare, as most people lose their employer-sponsored coverage when they retire.

Second, in 1983 Congress enacted legislation gradually increasing from sixty-five to sixty-seven the age at which Social Security recipients get a standard benefit—the so-called "full benefit age."[15] Some have suggested that this change justifies increasing the age of eligibility for Medicare to age sixty-seven as well. Increasing the age of eligibility for Medicare would probably marginally increase labor force participation and boost payroll and income tax collections. However, the direct reduction in Medicare spending would be surprisingly small—only about 6 percent (see table 4-2), because younger retirees incur much smaller health bills than do older retirees and raising the eligibility age has no effect on outlays for the non-elderly disabled.

In addition, these savings would be partly offset by increases in other federal outlays. Ineligibility for Medicare would push some sixty-five- to sixty-seven-year-olds into Medicaid and other government programs, notably those of the Veterans Administration. The increase in Medicaid enrollments would be particularly problematic for states, which have relatively inelastic revenue sources and operate under balanced budget requirements. An increase in the Medicare eligibility age would also push millions to seek private insurance coverage, but many have chronic illnesses—"preexisting conditions," in insurance jargon—that result in high premiums or denial of coverage. Were an increase in the Medicare eligibility age to come along without an increase in the actual age of retirement, all of these problems would be exacerbated.

Increased Medicare Cost Sharing

Requiring Medicare enrollees to pay more for care than they now do would lower federal outlays in two ways—by shifting costs from the government to the individual and by reducing individuals' use of health services by increasing the price that they have to pay. A major social experiment in which participants were exposed to varying deductibles provided evidence that the reductions in the use of care could be large.[16] The adverse health impacts from reduced use of health care services were small for most enrollees, but they were most notable for the disadvantaged. Whether the large cost savings and small health effects would carry over to the elderly and disabled populations is unclear, as both groups were excluded from the experiment; moreover, the health problems of the elderly differ greatly from those of the healthy, non-elderly population.

Medicare already requires considerable cost sharing by its enrollees. Part A, which covers hospital and skilled nursing facility stays, imposes higher deductibles and more cost sharing than most private plans and provides no protection for very lengthy hospital stays.[17] Enrollees must pay sizable premiums for Part B—Supplemental Medical Insurance (SMI)—which covers physicians' services, durable medical equipment, and the new drug benefit.[18] In 2003, Congress introduced income-related premiums for SMI for the first time in Medicare's history. Beginning in 2007, individuals and couples with incomes in excess of $80,000 and $160,000 respectively will have to pay premiums set at 35 to 80 percent of average premium cost. The top premiums will apply only when income exceeds $200,000 for individuals and $400,000 for couples. However, many people do not pay Part B premiums. About 33 percent of

Medicare-enrolled retirees have retiree coverage from their former employers that pays some or all deductibles, premiums, and copayments.[19] Other Medicare enrollees buy insurance themselves. And approximately 7.2 million elderly and disabled people are eligible for both Medicare and Medicaid, which pays most charges and covers certain services excluded from the Medicare benefits package—most notably, nursing home care.[20]

While raising the proportion of Medicare outlays paid by all enrollees would reduce both budget outlays and consumption of medical services, it would create two problems. First, increased premiums and charges for care could seriously burden all but upper-income elderly and disabled beneficiaries, especially if Social Security benefits are reduced.[21] Second, demand for preventive care, such as screening tests and maintenance therapy to slow the development of progressive conditions, seems to be sensitive to price. As a result, some analysts recommend providing such services outside deductibles, at little or no charge.

Other cost-sharing reforms should be considered. The various deductibles for different Medicare services could be replaced by a single deductible covering all services. Cost sharing for various services could be substantially increased, in combination with income-graduated waivers for low- and middle-income beneficiaries. A stop-loss provision should be added to Medicare to preclude the devastatingly large charges paid by some recipients under the current system.

The potential budget savings from such reforms should not be exaggerated. Typical elderly and disabled Medicare beneficiaries have modest incomes and few assets. For example, in 2002 only 15 percent of those over age sixty-five lived in households with incomes of $50,000 a year or more.[22] Large increases in cost sharing would threaten Medicare's basic purpose, unless they were limited to the minority of beneficiaries with high incomes.

New Medicare Purchasing Strategies

Medicare tries to limit costs by setting the price it will pay for various services. Many observers now believe that alternative systems could both lower costs and improve quality. Currently, for example, Medicare pays hospitals on the basis of each patient's primary and secondary diagnosis at admission and pays physicians for procedures performed. The system is enormously complicated to administer, with thousands of different prices; it also is virtually impossible to police fairly at a reasonable cost. For example, without intrusive and expensive administration, how is Medicare to know whether each physician or hospital correctly coded the services performed? For purposes of cost control, the physician payment system has an important additional shortcoming—it controls the price but not the quantity of services rendered. It thereby encourages the provision of low-benefit or even useless tests and procedures. Some observers believe that sizable savings could be achieved under alternative purchasing systems with different incentives.

PAY FOR INSURANCE, NOT CARE. Medicare now pays for services for 88 percent of beneficiaries, while 12 percent are enrolled in prepaid group plans. Medicare could instead pay a flat sum, adjusted for each patient's age and health status, to a health plan of the enrollee's choice—including HMOs, PPOs, point-of-service arrangements, or plans providing fee-for-service care. Under one possible arrangement, modeled on the Federal Employee Health Benefit Program (FEHBP), the federal government would contribute a flat amount equal to a fixed percentage of a weighted average of the premiums of the various plans participating. The current FEHBP share is 72 percent.

Because enrollees pay extra for plans whose premiums exceed the government's contribution, advocates of this approach maintain that they will tend to enroll in cost-effective plans, driving plans to compete to improve the quality of service and control costs. Critics express concern that Congress will not raise federal payments as fast as health costs increase, leading to erosion of Medicare coverage. Linking the federal payment to the cost of a basic package of health services rather than to costs—so-called "premium support"—might ameliorate this problem.[23] Critics of insurance vouchers or premium support also fear that numerous competing health plans would lack the leverage Medicare now has in securing low prices from providers.

SELECTIVE PURCHASING. Medicare now pays for care rendered by any willing provider for about 90 percent of current enrollees. Some observers argue that Medicare could lower costs and improve quality of care if it *selectively* purchased coverage, either from health plans or directly from providers. Favored vendors would be selected on the basis of cost and quality of services. Medicare enrollees would face additional charges if they chose a plan with high costs or of low quality. Incentives that might push insurers and providers to improve care and lower costs are more appealing to most people than stiff cost sharing at point of use, particularly for an elderly and disabled population, most of whom have modest income and few assets and many of whom lack the capacity or information to make good choices on their own.

Medicaid Modifications

Contrary to popular belief, Medicaid spends far more to support care for aged, blind, and disabled individuals than for poor mothers and their dependent children. Although the aged, blind, and disabled represented only 27 percent of Medicaid recipients in 2000, they accounted for 70 percent of program spending.[24] Thus the same demographic trends driving Medicare expenditures will also push up Medicaid outlays. Medicaid differs from Medicare in that a far larger share of its outlays go for nursing home benefits. Medicaid pays for 50 percent of nursing home care and 43 percent of total spending on long-term care.[25]

Medicaid is administered jointly with the states, most of which bear 40 to 50 percent of the costs. As a result, many changes to improve Medicaid efficiency are not entirely under federal control. Medicaid is the most rapidly growing component of state budgets. As the baby boom generation ages and eventually moves into the age brackets that make heavy use of nursing home services, Medicaid costs will threaten to overwhelm state budgets.

Unless enrollees become healthier or richer, federal Medicaid outlays can be cut in only five ways: by curtailing services, by buying services more cheaply or using them more efficiently, by encouraging people to buy private long-term care insurance, by reducing fraud, and by shifting costs to states.

CURTAILING SERVICES. Major restrictions on eligibility or covered services under Medicaid would directly undermine the program's goal of providing health care to the low-income population. Nor is significant cost sharing an option. Because Medicaid eligibility is based on lack of income or wealth, increasing charges would amount to denying services to enrollees. Nonetheless, because of severe fiscal pressures at the state level, governors are currently doing exactly that. Some states are proposing to pay only for primary and preventive care, leaving specialty care, diagnostic services, and hospitalization uncovered. Others are instituting premiums for at least some Medicaid enrollees.

BUYING SERVICES MORE CHEAPLY OR USING THEM MORE EFFICIENTLY. The second way to lower the growth of Medicaid spending is through new purchasing strategies. Medicaid now costs less than private insurance, after adjustments are made for coverage and patient characteristics, largely because Medicaid has stringently restricted fees. In addition, Medicaid costs have risen less in recent years than the costs of private care. Nonetheless, opportunities for additional economies exist. Medicaid participants continue to rely on emergency rooms for routine care that could be provided more effectively and economically in a physician's office. The lack of regular caregivers means that too often illnesses are not caught early and chronic conditions and disabilities are not adequately monitored, reducing the quality of care.[26] Whether fixing those problems would save money is less clear.

Several states have begun to buy health care at discounted prices for low-income populations from one or a small number of providers. Such contracts may incorporate quality indicators, such as reports that show whether the organization provides appropriate care in a timely fashion. States have also experimented with paying the employee's share of employer-sponsored health coverage for low-income workers and adding coverage when that provided by an employer plan is narrower than the Medicaid benefit package. This approach spares Medicaid the full cost of coverage. As with other supposedly cost-saving measures, such interventions are more likely to improve the quality of services than to cut their cost.

PRIVATE LONG-TERM CARE INSURANCE. The third way to lower Medicaid spending is to encourage people to buy long-term care insurance to protect themselves from nursing home costs, which currently run more than $60,000 a year for a semiprivate room offering custodial care.[27] Although some analysts see private long-term care insurance as the best hope for reducing the enormous projected growth in Medicaid spending on nursing home care, finding ways to induce people to buy and retain long-term care insurance has proven elusive.[28] Insurers have been loath to provide complete coverage because of uncertainty regarding service costs many years in the future. On the buyers' side, demand for long-term care insurance has been weak.

REDUCING FRAUD. Both Medicare and Medicaid pay large sums for services that are both expensive and hard to monitor, a combination that always breeds fraud. Medicare and Medicaid are not exceptional in this regard. So-called Medicaid mills have defrauded the program of millions in payment for needless procedures that were not, in fact, provided. For years, "up-coding," whereby providers bill for services that are more highly reimbursed than those that they actually provided, was generally acknowledged but rarely documented. The federal government has collected more than $12 billion in settlements from fraud cases since 1986, with the majority of those funds recovered from health care cases. Of $2.1 billion recovered in civil fraud claims in FY2003, $1.7 billion involved health care fraud—primarily against Medicare but more recently including substantial Medicaid settlements.[29]

SHIFTING COSTS TO THE STATES. The final way to rein in federal Medicaid spending is to shift costs to the states. Currently the federal government pays from 50 percent to 78 percent of state Medicaid service costs. In 2003 the Bush administration first proposed converting Medicaid from a matching grant to a block grant,[30] but the initiative was adamantly opposed by both Republican and Democratic governors, who recognized that states would face the full fiscal burden of rising enrollments. That risk is particularly acute during recessions, when applications increase and state revenues fall. Because of united opposition from the states, the administration did not reintroduce the block grant idea but instead floated the idea of capping payments per enrollee. This proposal provides the states some cushion against rising enrollments. They would still be forced to pay all of any increase in health costs above the cap, however, and they would be under heightened pressure to curtail benefits and limit enrollments.

Summary

There is no practicable way to estimate by how much the reforms described in this chapter would lower Medicare and Medicaid spending or health care outlays. Sizable reductions in the growth of government spending as a share of gross domestic product are doubtless possible. We believe, however, that the evidence shows conclusively that eliminating large increases in these budget shares is impossible without undermining the purpose of both programs and adversely affecting the health of elderly, disabled, and poor Americans. The largest reductions in government spending would result from increased cost sharing under Medicare, which makes sense for those who can afford it, and raising the age of eligibility, which might create more problems than it would solve. All of the measures presented here would take years to implement. Meanwhile, the population will be aging and using more health care per person, and physicians and other scientists will be developing new beneficial—and costly—forms of diagnosis and therapy. In the next section, we explore various ways in which the nation might adjust to the resulting cost increases.

Confronting Rising Health Costs: Three Budget Options

We turn now to three ways to deal with the huge projected increase in federal health care spending and its impact on the federal budget and on Medicare and Medicaid recipients. The same scenarios are also described in chapter 2, where their implications for other federal spending and the non-elderly population are further elaborated.

—Under the first scenario, we assume that the age of eligibility for Medicare remains sixty-five and that other aspects of the program are unchanged. We assume also that coverage and benefits under Medicare and Medicaid are unchanged and that health care costs continue to rise at the historical average of 2.5 percentage points a year faster than economic growth. Alternatively, some or all of the cost-reducing measures described earlier in this chapter could be introduced, with all of the savings used to bring Medicare coverage up to the standards of typical private insurance or to finance extended long-term care benefits. (This is the "maintaining the social contract" scenario in chapter 2.)

—The second scenario assumes that the growth of health care spending is somehow reduced from the historical average of 2.5 percentage points to 1 percentage point a year more than per capita GDP. Such a slowdown could occur in various ways. The Medicare eligibility age might be increased to seventy. Some combination of system reforms, such as those described earlier in this chapter, might be introduced. Or general health care rationing might slow the growth of all health care spending, public and private. We indicate the amount by which revenues would have to increase to pay for remaining health benefits. (This is the "investing in the future" scenario in chapter 2.)

—Under the third scenario, we assume that the share of gross domestic product devoted to Medicare and Medicaid increases solely because of demographic changes in the population. This scenario implies that per capita health care spending grows at the same rate as per capita income. We describe some of the program changes that such a cost constraint implies. (This is the "smaller government" scenario in chapter 2.)

Scenario 1: No Reduction in Growth of per Capita Health Costs

Under scenario 1, federal spending on Medicare and Medicaid will grow dramatically (see table 4-1). We assume that all of the increase would have to be covered by increased taxes. If growth of Medicare and Medicaid spending per beneficiary did not slow and if payroll and income taxes were used to cover the added costs of Medicare and Medicaid, it would be necessary to nearly double the Medicare payroll tax and increase all personal income tax collections by more than 70 percent to cover Medicare and Medicaid costs. (By 2040, payroll taxes would be two-and-a-half times higher and income tax collections would need to more than double.) Other possible ways of covering these increased costs are described in chapter 5.[31]

Scenario 2: Slowed Growth of Health Costs per Beneficiary

The first scenario makes clear that if growth of health care spending continues at past rates, massive tax increases are inescapable. We therefore suggest an approach that blends some program reductions with tax increases that, while formidable, are less extreme than those with option 1.

The second scenario is based on the assumption that the growth of per capita Medicare and Medicaid spending will moderately decelerate until the annual increase is just 1 percentage point more than the growth in wages, the same assumption used in projections by Medicare's actuaries. To achieve this slowdown will take aggressive action. Such actions will include most or all of the measures that various reformers have suggested and that we described above, including some increase in the age of eligibility for Medicare, increased cost sharing, selective purchasing, and the application of information technology. Even with such measures, it is unlikely that Medicare and Medicaid will be able to continue to provide essentially all beneficial care to those whom they serve. Increasing the age of eligibility for Medicare by five years would reduce spending by only 1.3 percent of GDP in 2030 and 1.5 percent in 2040. Medicare and Medicaid are likely to have to extend contracting with prepaid plans that not only have incentives to provide care efficiently but that also are prepared to ration care.

Medicare enrollees may be able to shoulder more cost sharing in the future than they can now to the extent that health savings accounts are adopted and people carry forward the unused balances in their accounts. Whether HSAs will be widely used is still unclear. If they are used, people may spend all or most of the funds deposited in such accounts during their working lives. And those who carry sizable balances forward are quite likely to reduce other forms of saving. For all of these reasons, the net effect of HSAs on the capacity of future Medicare beneficiaries to shoulder increased cost sharing is questionable.

If growth of per capita Medicare and Medicaid spending can be slowed to 1 percentage point more than GDP, federal spending on health care will still increase, as shown in table 4-1. Taxes would have to increase by 4 percent of gross domestic product by 2030 and 6 percent by 2040 just to cover added health care spending on Medicare and Medicaid. That increase makes no allowance for tax increases for other purposes—to balance the overall budget, to pay for added pension costs, to cover long-term care benefits beyond those now provided under Medicaid, or for military emergencies.

But a reduction in the growth of health care spending from 2.5 percentage points a year more than GDP to just 1 percentage point a year more would be a monumental achievement. It will demand vigorous action to promote cost-effective delivery of care and significant reductions in coverage.

Scenario 3: GDP and per Capita Health Care Spending Rise at the Same Rate

Under the third scenario, we assume that sufficient changes are made in Medicare and Medicaid to ensure that per beneficiary spending grows no faster than total national per capita income. Even so, Medicare and Medicaid will claim a growing share of government spending because the proportion of the population that is elderly and disabled is projected to grow.[32] If growth of per capita health spending did not exceed GDP growth, demography alone would be projected to increase federal Medicare and Medicaid expenditures from 4.2 percent of GDP in 2005 to 5.7 percent in 2030 and 6.2 percent in 2040.[33]

If per capita health costs continued to grow at historical rates, the share of GDP absorbed by federal health care spending could be held to these levels only by increasing the age of eligibility for Medicare from sixty-five to seventy-nine by 2030 and eighty-three by 2040. Many would find such increases in the age of eligibility unthinkable. As noted, even with such sharp increases in the age of eligibility, the total cost of Medicare as a share of gross domestic product would increase because the elderly and disabled will constitute a growing share of the total population.

Alternatively, deductibles, copayments, and coinsurance could be increased. This policy would shift costs now borne by Medicare to program beneficiaries and to the states, as higher cost sharing would push some people into Medicaid. In 2000, Medicare paid just under three-fifths of total personal health care spending of beneficiaries living in the community.[34] Whether that share will rise or fall depends in part on the character of medical advances and in part on policy. For example, the rapid increase in drug costs from 5.6 percent of personal health care spending in 1980 to 12.4 percent in 2003 increased out-of-pocket spending because Medicare did not cover outpatient drugs. With the passage of the Medicare Modernization Act of 2003, Medicare now covers some of those costs.

Policies that explicitly shift costs to enrollees would have two major effects. First, they would tend to reduce total health care spending. Second, they would increase the number of Medicare participants who also are eligible for Medicaid and who would turn to the Veterans Administration hospitals for care. The omission of the first effect understates budget savings; the omission of the second overstates savings. We ignore both such effects. Under this assumption, to hold the growth of per capita budget outlays on Medicare to that of per capita income, it would be necessary to lower the proportion of personal health care spending paid by Medicare from just under 60 percent to about 29 percent in 2030 and 23 percent in 2040.

Some combination of increases in the age of initial entitlement and cost sharing could also hold the growth in Medicare costs to growth resulting entirely from demographic shifts. Were growth of overall federal spending to be held to growth from demographic shifts, it would be necessary also to cut Medicaid coverage. If cuts in Medicaid spending are proportionately smaller than those in Medicare, holding growth of overall federal health care spending to what is attributable to growth of the population served would require even larger Medicare cuts than those indicated above. Even with the formidable cutbacks in coverage described above, federal health care spending would increase by 2 to 3 percent of GDP because of demographic forces alone.

The Rest of Health Care Spending

Nearly half of total health care spending now results from Medicare, Medicaid, and federal and state health programs for veterans and their families, and others.[35] Private health care spending will be affected less by population aging than will Medicare and Medicaid outlays. But private health care spending will be subject to the same upward pressures from technology. As shown in table 4-3, continued growth at historical rates indicates that total health care spending will absorb more than one-fourth of gross domestic product by 2030 and more than one-third by 2040. Increased private costs for care will come on top of the sharply higher taxes to support benefits for dependent populations. Under those circumstances, we anticipate that pressures to ration care for the entire

Table 4-3. *Projection of National Health Care Spending*
as a Percent of GDP under Two Scenarios[a]

Year	Historical trend scenario (percent)	Slowed growth scenario (percent)
2005	15.6[b]	15.6[b]
2010	17.3[b]	17.3[b]
2020	21.6	19.8
2030	27.6	21.9
2040	35.2	24.1

a. The historical trend scenario assumes that Medicare and Medicaid cost growth exceeds GDP by 2.5 percent a year. The slowed growth scenario assumes that Medicare and Medicaid cost growth exceeds GDP by 1 percent a year.

b. Estimates of the Centers for Medicare and Medicaid Services (www.cms.hhs.gov/statistics/nhe/ [March 17, 2005]) and authors' calculations.

population will intensify. The idea of health care rationing now offends most Americans. However, an ever-tightening squeeze on the capacity of Americans to afford goods and services other than health care may well persuade them that health care rationing, though very difficult and highly controversial, is less repugnant than the alternatives. The challenge is to develop ways to place systemwide limits on access to health care services in both the public and private sectors that have a rationale that the public can support.

How Do We Get from Here to There?

The United States can restrict health expenditures in three ways. It can limit the quantity of care demanded by raising the cost of care at the time of illness. It can slow the advance of technology. Or it can limit supply by restricting the use of available technologies.

The United States already rations care to those who are not well insured and do not have the means to pay for care. The 45 million people without health insurance, for example, consume on average only a little more than half of the health care services that insured people use. Health insurance could be changed so that it pays only for costs of care that exceed a high deductible. Two decades ago a major social experiment demonstrated that increasing the cost of care significantly reduced the quantity of care demanded. Proponents of requiring patients to pay more claim that doing so would also lower prices. Exposing patients to increased charges would surely lower the *level* of spending, but it is unlikely to reduce the *growth* of spending unless it slows the pace of technological advancement, an outcome that would probably lower over-all social welfare. Hopes that increasing patient charges would lower prices may be unrealistic because individuals would be less able than large groups to bargain for discounts. Most savings would result from services forgone.

The second approach would reduce growth of health care expenditures by directly controlling the principal engine of growth, the development of new medical technology, by limiting support for medical research. This approach would be of only limited efficacy because the United States is the home of much but not all medical research. Furthermore, some U.S. research is driven by the quest for profit and therefore would be hard for public policy to control. More telling is that such controls would reduce general welfare. Medical research has produced total benefits far greater than its cost, even if considerable waste occurs at the margin.[36]

The third approach is the most promising—to limit the supply of care by requiring care to be justified by "evidence-based" research. Total expenditures would be limited by private or public regulation. Funds would be allocated to services that produce a level of benefits per dollar spent that exceeds some specified threshold. This approach is conceptu-ally straightforward but formidably difficult to implement.[37] Medical knowledge of what technologies produce the greatest medical benefits in particular cases is lacking for many—perhaps most—conditions.

We are not confident about which approach to limiting growth of health care expenditures will—or should—be used. The nation is likely to try some combination of all three approaches. That it can avoid all of them seems unlikely.

Notes

1. Kevin Murphy and Robert Topel, eds., *Measuring the Gains from Medical Research: An Economic Approach* (University of Chicago Press, 2003); David M. Cutler and Mark McClellan, "Is Technological Change in Medicine Worth

It?" *Health Affairs* 20, no. 5 (2001): 11–29; Ernst Berndt and others, "Medical Care Prices and Output," in *The Handbook of Health Economics,* vol. 1A, edited by Anthony Culyer and Joseph Newhouse (Amsterdam: Elsevier, 2000), pp. 119–80.

2. Uwe E. Reinhardt, Peter S. Hussey, and Gerard F. Anderson, "U.S. Health Care Spending in an International Context," *Health Affairs* 23, no. 3 (2004): 11.

3. For a careful yet readily accessible review of recent developments, see John Potts and William B. Schwartz, "The Impact of the Revolution in Biomedical Research on Life Expectancy by 2050," in *Coping with Methuselah,* edited by Henry J. Aaron and William B. Schwartz (Brookings, 2003).

4. The automobile and the airplane lowered the price per mile of moving human beings and goods but increased total spending on transportation. Computers reduced the price of performing simple arithmetic operations but increased total spending on computation. Low computation costs in turn led to the use of computers in performing tasks for which no one had ever dreamed of using them. Movies and later television and cassette and DVD recordings reduced the price of seeing dramas, comedies, and musicals, but they increased outlays on entertainment. Millions who had lacked access to live concerts and stage performances or the means to attend them could enjoy a facsimile performance in one of thousands of theaters across the country or in their homes for a fraction of the cost of the real thing.

5. Cutler and McClellan, "Is Technological Change Worth It?"; Jonathan Skinner and John Wennberg, "How Much Is Enough? Efficiency and Medicare Spending in the Last Six Months of Life," in *The Changing Hospital Industry: Comparing Not-for-Profit and For-Profit Hospitals,* edited by David Cutler (University of Chicago Press, 2000). More generally, see "The Dartmouth Atlas of Health Care 1999" (www.dartmouthatlas.org/atlaslinks/99atlas.php [March 7, 2005]).

6. Studies document rates of inappropriate care in Germany, the Netherlands, Spain, and Great Britain similar to those reported for the United States. J. G. Lambert and others, "To Stay or Not to Stay: The Assessment of Appropriate Hospital Stay: A Dutch Report," *International Journal for Quality in Health Care* 14, no. 1 (2002): 55–67. Oliver Sangha and others, "Metric Properties of the Appropriateness Evaluation Protocol and Predictors of Inappropriate Hospital Use in Germany: An Approach Using Longitudinal Patient Data," *International Journal for Quality in Health Care* 14, no. 6 (2002): 483–92; Carlos Moya-Ruiz, Salvador Peiro, and Ricard Meneu, "Effectiveness of Feedback to Physicians in Reducing Inappropriate Use of Hospitalization: A Study in a Spanish Hospital," *International Journal for Quality in Health Care* 14, no. 4 (2002): 305–12; G. J. Elwyn and N. C. H. Stott, "Avoidable Referrals? Analysis of 170 Consecutive Referrals to Secondary Care," *British Medical Journal* 309 (September 3, 1994): 576–78.

7. Barbara Starfield, for example, attributed 225,000 deaths to medical treatments with various "iatrogenic causes" in "Is US Health Really the Best in the World?" *Journal of the American Medical Association* 284 (July 26, 2000): pp. 483–85. This would attribute 9.3 percent of deaths to iatrogenic causes, making

that the third-highest cause of death, after heart disease and cancer. Of those deaths, however, 106,000 were due to adverse reactions to medications for which there was no previous indication of a risk factor. Another 80,000 deaths were due to "nosocomial" infections (those acquired during hospital stays), which do not always reflect avoidable errors; in some cases, they reflect a natural risk of infection in hospitals, where patients are exposed to many germs. "How Common Are Medical Mistakes?" (www.wrongdiagnosis.com/mistakes/common.htm [March 8, 2005]).

8. A recent study indicates that while increases in malpractice settlements account for little of the growth in premiums and malpractice costs do not materially change the number of practicing physicians, increased malpractice liability may somewhat increase the use of such screening procedures as mammography, so-called defensive medicine. Katherine Baicker and Amitabh Chandra, "The Effect of Malpractice Liability on the Delivery of Health Care," Working Paper 10709 (Cambridge, Mass.: National Bureau of Economic Research, August 2004) (www.nber.org/papers/w10709 [March 8, 2005]).

9. Mark A. Schuster, Elizabeth A. McGlynn, and Robert H. Brook, "How Good Is the Quality of Health Care in the United States?" *Milbank Quarterly* 76, no. 4 (1998): 517–63.

10. Institute of Medicine, *Crossing the Quality Chasm: A New Health System for the 21st Century* (Washington: National Academy Press, 2001), p.228.

11. John Wennberg, Elliott Fisher, and Jonathan Skinner, "Geography and the Debate over Medicare Reform," *Health Affairs* 21 (Supplement): W97–W114; Elliott Fisher and others, "Variations in the Longitudinal Efficiency of Academic Medical Centers," *Health Affairs* web exclusive, October 7, 2004 (www.health affairs.org).

12. Peter McMenamin, "Dr. McCoy to Sickbay: Not 'Stat' but with All Deliberate Speed," May 19, 2004. McMenamin, a health economist based in Silver Spring, Maryland, lists a number of problems with the conversion to digital records. Implementing electronic records will take a large investment in translating old notes. It will take sophisticated software to assist physicians in sifting through the mountains of data that constitute typical medical records. Such software is not fully developed and will depend on advances in artificial intelligence, the feasibility of which remains in question. If these advances prove feasible, electronic records will prevent medical errors that are both costly and tragic, whether they eventually save money or not. Adequate methods of preserving privacy and accurately identifying individuals remain to be addressed. Conversion to digital records may ultimately lower costs, but claimed savings are not yet well documented and will take years to yield returns.

13. For a detailed explanation of HSAs, see Henry J. Aaron, "HSAs—The 'Sleeper' in the Medicare Bill," *Tax Notes,* February 23, 2004, pp. 1025–30.

14. Women could claim Social Security benefits as early as age sixty-two starting in 1956; men, after 1961.

15. Implementation of this change was delayed, however, so that the first affected workers were those turning age sixty-two in 2000. They were eligible to

receive full benefits at age sixty-five and two months. Only in 2022 will the full benefits age reach age sixty-seven for workers turning age sixty-two. Annual Statistical Supplement to the Social Security Bulletin, 2003 (Social Security Administration), table 2.A20 (www.ssa.gov/policy/docs/statcomps/supplement/2003/2a20-2a28.html#table2.a20 [March 22, 2005]).

16. Emmett Keeler, "Effects of Cost Sharing on Use of Medical Services and Health" (RAND Corporation, 1992) (www.rand.org/publications/RP/RP1114/RP1114.pdf [March 8, 2005]). Subjects enrolled in a plan with a $1,000 deductible (in 1975–81 dollars) consumed medical care costing 34 percent less than did those in a plan under which all care was free. Those who faced 25 percent cost sharing up to a $1,000 stop-loss level consumed care costing 19 percent less than those under the free-care plan. Translating those results into estimates of the impact of increased Medicare cost sharing on use is problematic because of general and health care price inflation, the exclusion of the elderly from the experiment, and differences in cost sharing and services covered in the experiment.

17. Hospital insurance requires patients to pay a deductible of $912 in 2005; copayments of $228 a day for hospital stays of sixty-one to ninety days and $456 a day for an additional sixty days of coverage during the patient's lifetime; and all costs for more extended hospital stays. Medicare imposes additional charges for the use of skilled nursing facilities and does not limit out-of-pocket payments. Patients could be forced to pay as much as $35,112 under Part A before Medicare stops paying altogether.

18. The annual premium for Part B is $938; the annual deductible is $110. Medicare enrollees also have to pay an annual premium estimated to be $420 to qualify for the Medicare drug benefit. If they enroll, they face a deductible of $250 and costs ranging from 5 percent to 100 percent of additional drug outlays, depending on how much they spend. A person with $3,000 in drug outlays, for example, would pay $1,920 in premiums and coinsurance.

19. Patricia Neuman, *The State of Retiree Health Benefits: Historical Trends and Future Uncertainties,* testimony to the Senate Special Committee on Aging," 108th Cong., 2nd. sess., May 17, 2004. Of the 5.8 million retirees between ages fifty-five and sixty-four, 57 percent (3.3 million) have retiree health coverage.

20. Brian Bruen and John Holahan, "Shifting the Cost of Dual Eligibles: Implications for States and the Federal Government" (Washington: Henry J. Kaiser Family Foundation, November 2003). For other exceptions, see "Medicare Cost Sharing and Premium Amounts" (www.cms.hhs.gov/publications/trusteesreport/2004/secivc.asp [March 8, 2005]).

21. Part B premiums are deducted from Social Security benefits before checks are mailed. According to estimates of the Center for Retirement Research, Medicare premiums claimed 6 percent of average Social Security benefits in 2000 and are projected to absorb nearly 11 percent of benefits by 2020. For retirees with low earnings histories, Medicare premiums take up an even larger share of benefits.

22. Social Security Administration, *Income of the Aged Chartbook 2001* (2003).

23. Premium support could raise other problems. How should the included set of services be adjusted as technology advances? How should the payment made on behalf of each enrollee be adjusted for age and health status? How should the design and marketing of plans be regulated to ensure that the elderly, many of whom are frail or mentally impaired, can understand the various offerings and choose intelligently among them? The term "premium support" was coined by Henry J. Aaron and Robert R. Reischauer, "The Medicare Reform Debate: What Is the Next Step?" *Health Affairs* 14, no. 4 (1995): 8–30.

24. Total spending on the aged, blind, and disabled was $117.2 billion; $44.5 billion was spent on other identified beneficiaries. Committee on Ways and Means, House of Representatives, *2004 Green Book,* table 15–17 (http://frweb-gate.access.gpo.gov/cgi-bin/useftp.cgi?IPaddress=162.140.64.88&filename=wm006_15.pdf&directory=/disk2/wais/data/108_green_book [March 8, 2005]).

25. Ellen O'Brien and Risa Elias, "Medicaid and Long Term Care" (Washington: Henry J. Kaiser Family Foundation, May 2004).

26. Several states are developing disease and case management programs to cope with this problem. Advocates claim they will improve health outcomes and lower costs by making sure that patients take prescribed medications, monitoring indicators that show whether chronic illnesses are under control, referring patients to appropriate medical specialists, coordinating care and developing individualized treatment plans, and involving relatives in patients' care.

27. MetLife Mature Market Institute, "The MetLife Market Survey of Nursing Home and Home Care Costs" (September 2004).

28. Several states have introduced programs to encourage people to purchase private long-term care insurance. For people who purchase a qualifying long-term care policy, states waive the requirement that they must completely spend down their assets in order to qualify for Medicaid. On retention, see Paul E. McNamara and Nayoung Lee (2004), "Long-Term Care Insurance Policy Dropping in the U.S. from 1996 to 2000: Evidence and Implications for Long-Term Care Financing," *Geneva Papers on Risk and Insurance: Issues and Practice* 29, no. 4 (October 2004): 640–51.

29. U.S. Department of Justice, "Justice Department Civil Fraud Recoveries Total $2.1 Billion for FY 2003: False Claims Act Recoveries Exceed $12 Billion since 1986," November 10, 2003.

30. Cindy Mann, Melanie Nathanson, and Edwin Park, "Administration's Medicaid Proposal Would Shift Fiscal Risks to States," Center on Budget and Policy Priorities, April 22, 2003 (www.cbpp.org/4-1-03health.htm [March 8, 2005]).

31. If Medicare hospital insurance continues to be financed largely by payroll taxes, the payroll tax rate would have to increase from its current 2.9 percent of all earnings in covered employment to 5.6 percent in 2030 and 7.2 percent in 2040. In addition, general revenues would have to be dedicated to Part B of Medicare and to Medicaid. An additional 6.5 percent of gross domestic product would be needed by 2030 and 10 percent by 2040. For comparison, the personal and corporation income taxes currently yield 9 percent of gross domestic product.

32. Growth of Social Security outlays can be used to gauge the impact of demography alone, as benefits are automatically adjusted for wage growth. Official estimates indicate that Social Security costs as a share of GDP will grow from 4.28 percent of GDP in 2005 to 6.31 percent in 2030 and 6.54 percent on 2040. These estimates include the effects of legislated reductions in benefits subsequent to 2005 of about 7 percent by 2030 and about 8 percent by 2040. Thus demography alone can be expected to increase the share of GDP devoted to Medicare by roughly three-fifths by 2030 and roughly two-thirds by 2040.

33. The GDP shares in 2030 and 2040 allow for expenditures under the Medicare drug benefit that begin only in 2006.

34. AARP, "What Share of Beneficiaries' Total Health Care Costs Does Medicare Pay?" (http://research.aarp.org/health/dd78_costs.html [March 8, 2005]). In 2000 Medicare paid 59.2 percent of total personal health care expenditures; Medicaid, 5.5 percent; private insurance, 13.3 percent; out-of-pocket funds, 16.9 percent; and other, 5.1 percent. The Medicare share was lower and the Medicaid share higher for institutionalized patients.

35. Data from the Centers on Medicare and Medicaid, 2004, "National Health Expenditures by Type of Service and Source of Funds, 2003" (www.cms. hhs.gov/statistics/nhe/default.asp#download [March 8, 2005]).

36. See note 1.

37. See Henry J. Aaron and William B. Schwartz, *Can We Say No? The Challenge of Health Care Rationing* (Brookings, 2005, forthcoming).

5

Tax Policy Solutions

WILLIAM G. GALE AND
C. EUGENE STEUERLE

Taxes play a central role in long-term fiscal issues. The *level* of revenue collected must ultimately be sufficient to finance the chosen level of spending. Likewise, the *structure* of tax policy has far-ranging effects on the economy, similar to the structure of spending programs. This chapter is a guide to reforms that, in our view, could improve the structure of taxes and could align revenue levels with different chosen levels of spending.[1]

The fundamental goals of tax policy appear to be widely accepted: taxes should be simple, transparent, stable, and fair; encourage economic prosperity; impose minimal costs on the economy; raise the revenue needed to finance chosen spending levels; yet respect individuals' freedom and privacy. Nevertheless, this broad consensus barely scratches the surface of real tax issues. People often have different ideas of what each goal means: fairness, for example, is in the eyes of the beholder. They may disagree on the best way to achieve a goal. Is the most effective way to increase growth to reduce the budget deficit, to cut tax rates, or to invest in education and health? Most important, they may disagree about what to do when the goals are in conflict with each other—for example, what to do if a particular proposal raises the progressivity of the tax system but also reduces work effort.

As a result of these differences, changes in tax policy tend to be controversial. Nonetheless, the nation has no option but to align revenue and spending levels in the long run, and we believe that tax structure could be durably improved at any given revenue level.

Background

The federal government raises revenue from four main sources: the personal income tax, payroll taxes, the corporate income tax, and estate and gift taxes. Over the past fifty years, the personal income tax has been the workhorse, in terms of raising revenues and providing progressivity. Payroll taxes have risen substantially over the last several decades and are now the second largest revenue source. Most households pay more in payroll taxes than in income taxes. Payroll taxes are earmarked to pay for social insurance benefits; the taxes themselves are regressive, but the overall effect of the programs, including taxes and benefits, is progressive. Corporate tax revenues have fallen sharply as a share of GDP over the past fifty years. The estate and gift taxes raise small amounts of revenues but are a key element of the progressivity of the federal tax system.

As described in chapter 1, the personal income tax and estate tax are currently in a state of flux because since 2001 numerous tax provisions have been passed on a temporary basis. Under current law, all of these recent tax cuts will expire by the end of 2010.

In 2004 the federal government collected revenues of $1.9 trillion. At 16.3 percent of GDP, revenues were at their lowest share of the economy since 1951. As shown in chapter 1, under the baseline that would make almost all of the recent tax cuts permanent and avoid big tax increases due to an alternative minimum tax (AMT), revenues in 2015 are projected to be only 17 percent of GDP, less than the average of 18.2 percent between 1960 and 2000. Thus as the nation heads into a lengthy period of expanded budgetary pressures, revenues are likely to be running well below their historical share of GDP.

After 2015, the revenue picture improves only slightly. The adjusted baseline implies revenues of 20 percent of GDP by 2030. Although this would be close to the highest revenue level since World War II, it would still be far below projected spending equal to about 27 percent of GDP in 2030 under current policies (see chapter 2). This suggests the need either for very large cuts in spending, very large tax increases, or some of both, relative to the adjusted baseline.

How to distribute such taxes equitably among households—within and across generations—is both controversial and laden with judgment. There is widespread agreement that a fair tax should provide "equal treatment"; that is, households or individuals that are in equivalent economic situations should be treated equivalently. In practice, however, it is sometimes difficult to reach agreement on what constitutes an equivalent economic situation.

Most people also believe a fair tax should be progressive, though there is sharp disagreement about *how* progressive taxes should be. Progressivity refers to the extent to which the ratio of taxes paid to income (or some other measure of economic capacity or well-being) rises as income (or another measure of capacity) rises. The overall progressivity of government policy, however, is determined by both taxes and expenditures. For low- and moderate-income households, the redistribution achieved through government spending may swamp tax-induced redistributions. Thus the current and projected budget deficits, which are crimping federal spending for low- and middle-income families, threaten to make the overall system more regressive.

In general, the tax system should do as little damage as possible to the level and composition of economic activity.[2] Uneven rates across activities or assets encourage people to choose projects with inferior economic returns but favorable tax treatment over projects with stronger economic returns but less favorable tax rules. This leads to a misallocation of resources and an unambiguous decline in economic well-being. Several areas of the federal tax code stand out in this regard, in particular the favorable treatment of housing and the varying treatment of different forms of business income.

Changes in tax levels and rates have two sets of effects on the economy. First, they directly affect economic decisions. Lower marginal tax rates, for example, can stimulate work, saving, investment, and risk taking. (On the other hand, to the extent that tax cuts reduce tax liabilities without affecting marginal rates, people will feel richer and are likely to reduce work effort and similar economic activity.) Available evidence suggests that although these effects can be large when tax rates are very high, in general the broad impacts on labor supply, saving, investment, or risk taking are modest when the rates themselves are lower.

Second, tax cuts have indirect effects on the economy. Without offsetting reductions in spending, tax cuts raise the budget deficit, which reduces public saving. When national saving—the sum of private and public saving—falls, the future income of American households is reduced. In many cases the negative effect from increasing the budget deficit outweighs the positive direct effect of a tax cut.[3] In short, whether tax increases support or hamper economic growth depends on how they are designed and financed. The evidence suggests that as long as tax rates remain in a moderate range, small differences in marginal tax rates by themselves exert only modest influences on work, saving, and entrepreneurship, while sustained budget deficits reduce growth.

Currently, the highest marginal rates are faced by poor and middle-income households, especially when children are present. The reason is that benefits from many government programs phase out quite sharply as income increases, and hence effectively "tax" any increase in income earned by such families.

Besides affecting incentives to work and save, high tax rates also give taxpayers incentives to avoid (legally) and evade (illegally) taxes. Thus, lower rates can encourage taxpayers to report more of their income and to restructure their activities to include more taxable activity and less untaxed activity. The magnitude of these effects is open to question, but their importance is heightened by an estimated "tax gap"—taxes that should be paid but are not—in excess of $300 billion per year.

Although there is near-unanimous agreement that the federal tax system is too complex, taxes seem to become more complicated every year. Some complexity is an unavoidable by-product of trying to achieve other policy goals, such as greater equity or better enforcement. Nevertheless, we believe that much of it could be eliminated without loss of important social policy objectives. The political process, however, often ignores the costs of complexity in new legislation and then constrains simplification efforts for fear of creating losers.

Replacing the Current System

One approach to dealing with the problems described above is to jettison most of the current tax code and start over with a completely new system. Advocates of fundamental tax reform claim that it could boost growth, slash tax burdens, simplify compliance, and eliminate the Internal Revenue Service. Unfortunately, a more realistic assessment of the problem must acknowledge that all taxes involve some complexity and require a government agency to handle returns, audit taxpayers, and deter cheating—and no tax will satisfy all taxpayers.

In recent years, several consumption-based taxes have been proposed as alternatives to the existing system. Under a national retail sales tax (NRST), a single tax rate would apply to all sales by businesses to households. (Sales between businesses and between households would not be taxed.) Under a value added tax (VAT), each business would pay tax on the difference between its total sales, whether to consumers or to other businesses, and its purchases from other businesses, including investment. Thus the incremental value at each stage of production is subject to tax. Cumulated over all stages of production, the tax base just equals the value of final sales by businesses to consumers—that is, it is the same, in theory, as under an NRST.

The flat tax, whose name was originally developed by Hoover Institution scholars Robert Hall and Alvin Rabushka, is simply a two-part VAT: the business tax base would be exactly like the VAT, except that businesses would be allowed deductions not only for purchases from other businesses but also for cash wage and salary payments and employer pension contributions.[4] Individuals would then pay tax on wages, salaries, and pension income that exceeded personal and dependent exemptions. Businesses and individuals would be taxed at a single flat rate. Under the "jettison the income tax" approach, the NRST, the VAT, and the flat tax would replace the current convoluted income tax base with a consumption base, replace the current graduated rate structure with a single tax rate (or at least a single positive rate), and eliminate almost all tax credits and deductions.[5]

As replacements for the current system, the consumption tax proposals made to date are unlikely to function all that simply or to be politically acceptable, although they might sound appealing relative to an unreformed income tax. In the national retail sales tax, the tax rate required to replace income and payroll taxes and maintain current government programs would be on the order of 40 or 50 percent. Likewise, realistic versions of the flat tax—including measures of transition relief; allowances for individual deductions for charity, large health payments, and state taxes; and business deductions for health insurance and taxes— would require rates of over 30 percent just to replace the personal and corporate income taxes.

In addition, both systems would provide large tax cuts for the wealthiest households and make up the revenue with tax increases for low- and middle-income households. Finally, international experience suggests that retail sales tax rates above 10 percent stretch the limits of enforcement. The flat tax would also face significant avoidance problems at the business level, both because it treats some cash flows (such as interest and dividend payments) differently from others (such as purchases of goods and services) and because firms and tax advisers have devised very clever ways to "relabel" such flows to gain tax advantages.

Piecemeal Moves toward Flat Consumption Taxes

Completely replacing the existing system would entail enormous administrative, legislative, and economic upheavals. This has led some to advocate step-by-step replacement of particular features of the tax code, with the goal of converting progressive taxes on income and wealth into a flat tax on consumption. Such changes typically include reductions in marginal income tax rates, especially for high-income households; increases in contribution limits for tax-preferred savings accounts; expensing (immediate write-offs) of business investment, rather than depreciation over time; repeal of the estate tax; and a reduction in dividends and capital gains taxes. Many of these changes are reflected in the Bush administration's recent rate cuts, dividend and capital gains tax cuts, expansions of contribution limits to IRAs and 401(k)s, and temporary "bonus depreciation" provisions. The administration has also proposed vast expansions in the contribution limits for tax-free savings accounts.

The problem is that these changes do not add up to a well-defined tax system. In theory, an efficient consumption tax would (a) collect adequate revenues to cover expenditures over time and avoid reducing national saving through higher government deficits; (b) broaden the base to reduce interference in the economy; (c) tax already-existing capital—that is, concentrate any revenue relief on new saving or investment; and (d) treat interest income and expense in a consistent manner. But the piecemeal proposals and legislative changes of recent years fail all four tests. They (a) reduce government saving, and likely national saving; (b) do not broaden the base; (c) reduce taxes on existing capital; and (d) increase the difference in the tax treatment of interest income and expense.

Some advocates of piecemeal reform downplay such concerns, arguing that the perfect is the enemy of the good. But our underlying point is that the system that emerges has many of the worst features of *both* the earlier tax system and a fundamentally reformed system. First, the administration's tax cuts accompanied an expansion in expenditure, leading to deficits that may reduce long-term economic growth. Second, there will be no efficiency gains from broadening the base if no base-broadening occurs. Third, efficiency is reduced because windfall gains—for example, from cuts in taxes on dividends and capital gains—raise the return to old investments without inducing more saving. Fourth, there will be efficiency losses from increases in taxpayers' ability to shelter income without saving more if differences between the taxation of capital income and capital expense become larger—that is, if tax preferences for deposits to accounts are expanded but interest deductions are retained.

By excluding returns to capital from taxation but not returns to labor, this system shifts the burden of taxation to low- and moderate-income households, which receive the bulk of their income in the form of wages. And the system would also allow interest deductions, which would allow high-income taxpayers to shelter some of their wages, so that the tax burden would fall even more heavily on the wages of low- and middle-income households.

Reforming the Current System

There are numerous areas where the current tax system could be changed. This section discusses some of the major possibilities.

Deal with the Expiring Tax Cuts

The most immediate tax questions facing the country are to what extent the administration's recent tax cuts, including some not yet implemented, are to be made permanent, and if so, how they would be financed. Ultimately, tax cuts must be paid for either with spending cuts or other tax increases. To date, however, no leader in either political party has indicated how these and other recent deficit-increasing measures will be paid for. The administration has actually proposed budget rules that would allow Congress to pass legislation to make the tax cuts permanent without showing any cost relative to a "current law baseline." In fact, making the tax cuts permanent would reduce revenues after 2011 by about 2 percent of GDP.

If these tax cuts were financed with spending cuts, the required reductions in spending would be enormous. In 2015, for example, if Social Security, Medicare, Medicaid, homeland security, defense, and net interest were all off limits, a 50 percent reduction in all other government spending would be required to cover the revenue loss from having made the tax cuts permanent. For the tax cuts to be financed by tax increases, a majority in Congress and the president would have to commit themselves to tax reform that increased net revenues rather than reform that is revenue neutral. To the extent that insufficient tax increases or spending cuts occur, the tax cuts would be temporarily financed by borrowing. This postpones, but does not avoid, the ultimate need to cut spending or raise taxes. Moreover, borrowing to finance tax cuts that have not been paid for will reduce long-term growth, according to studies by a variety of experts and also the Congressional Budget Office. Slower growth would eventually create an even bigger gap to fill. In short, whether the tax cuts are made permanent is as much a first-order economic issue as are the very large scheduled increases in spending discussed in previous chapters.

Broaden the Base

A central goal of tax reform should be to define the tax base, whether income or consumption, as consistently, broadly, and simply as possible. More evenhanded taxation of different forms of income or consumption means that taxpayers in similar circumstances are treated similarly and one type of activity is not favored arbitrarily over another. Eliminating special provisions simplifies the system, and the expanded base raises revenues that can be used to reduce tax rates or fund government programs.

The tax reform enacted in 1986 cut back on more than $200 billion a year in tax exclusions, deductions, and credits, thus allowing government to operate with much lower statutory tax rates, yet retaining the progressivity of the system. Current tax subsidies total hundreds of billions of dollars per year. They must be addressed in any reform.

Although there are literally hundreds of special, targeted tax breaks in the tax system, the largest tax subsidies are for health, housing, saving for retirement or other purposes—each of which receive benefits in excess of $100 billion per year.[6] Other tax subsidies provide earnings supplements for poor and moderate-income workers or encourage charitable giving, research, investment, energy, production or efficiency, and environmental goals. In short, the bulk of the revenue loss is due to social and economic policies that provide benefits for large numbers of people. Many of these provisions have been present almost since the inception of the income tax, in 1913.

Nonetheless, we believe these provisions are often designed in ways that are ineffective, inequitable, and target-inefficient.[7] They largely subsidize activity that would have occurred anyway. They complicate tax filing and enforcement. They erode the tax base, requiring higher tax rates than would otherwise be necessary. They are regressive, giving bigger benefits to high-income than low-income filers. Finally, they hide subsidies that would be obvious if these same provisions were spending programs. Imagine that instead of a mortgage interest deduction, we had a program called "mortgage assistance," in which taxpayers earned an "entitlement" equal to their annual interest payment times their tax rate. Anyone whose entitlement was below a certain threshold, say $6,000, would receive nothing. Anyone whose entitlement exceeded the threshold would receive this amount in cash. Such a program would be decried as wasteful and a sop to the rich. Yet it works in much the same way as the mortgage interest deduction. Similarly, additional amounts spent each year on the major health tax subsidy—the exclusion of employer-provided insurance from taxable earnings—likely increase health expenditures, which in turn leads to an increase in the number of uninsured, which in turn leads to higher Medicaid costs.

Exclusions, deductions, and exemptions provide different subsidies to taxpayers in different brackets. This makes sense if the purpose of the deduction is to adjust the measure of income for ability to pay or to net expenses against gross income. But if the goal is to subsidize some group or activity, this design often makes less sense. A tax credit (or a deduction at a common rate) would provide the same marginal incentive for each household. Proposals along these lines could be designed to minimize revenue loss, dampen regressivity, and improve other aspects of existing subsidies.

Reform Incentives for Saving

Similar arguments apply to the current structure of tax incentives for saving. The revenue loss from retirement saving incentives alone is greater than personal saving in the United States, and although both these measures—lost revenues and personal saving—have limitations, the comparison reveals how little net saving such tax breaks are creating. As a result, the enormous (and expensive) efforts over the past twenty-five years to stimulate private saving by providing numerous tax incentives for *contributions* to particular accounts (which is quite different from new "saving") appear not to have been very successful in raising overall private saving, and even less successful in raising national saving, the sum of private and public saving.

Part of the problem is that the accounts do not subsidize saving, which requires a reduction in consumption spending and current living standards. Instead, they merely subsidize deposits (or contributions) into an account. These contributions can be made in many "painless" ways that do not involve reducing one's standard of living. High-income, high-wealth households are the most able to make such painless contributions, drawing from income they would have saved anyway, assets they already have saved, or borrowed money. As a result, limiting deductions for deposits when interest deductions are taken would help solve part of the problem. Another part of the problem is that the immediate incentive to contribute—as measured by the tax deductions that are allowed—is largest for these same high-income households.

The best way to raise saving may lie in using existing accounts better, rather than in raising contribution limits to IRAs or creating new accounts. Encouraging automatic enrollment and automatic escalation of contributions over time in existing 401(k) accounts is a primary example. The evidence suggests this would raise contribution rates among low- and moderate-income workers who are less likely to be using the accounts as tax shelters. Encouraging people to save their tax refunds or allowing automatic payroll deductions for individual retirement accounts would have similar effects. We believe that these moves—which are probably legal now but could be facilitated by legislative clarification—would have a much more positive impact on saving and well-being in retirement than piecemeal and inconsistent moves toward a consumption tax.

Along the same lines, expanding and making permanent the saver's credit would be an effective way to raise contributions among low- and middle-income taxpayers, who often have very little in the way of financial assets for retirement. The saver's credit provides a nonrefundable government matching contribution for individual contributions to 401(k) and IRA plans. The match rate declines as individual income rises. This tends to reverse the upside-down structure of existing saving incentives, which give larger deductions to higher-income households. Although expanding the saver's credit would entail a revenue cost, we believe that, per dollar of cost, it could do more to raise both private and national saving.

Fix the Alternative Minimum Tax

Under current law, roughly 30 million households will face the AMT by 2010; 42 million taxpayers will face the tax by 2015 if the 2001 and 2003 tax cuts are made permanent. As a result of this expansion, the efficiency, equity, transparency, and simplicity of the tax system are all threatened. Simply repealing the AMT, however, would dramatically reduce federal revenues and would encourage tax sheltering.

A better solution would be to fold the features of the AMT that are desirable, specifically those that close down aggressive tax sheltering, into the regular income tax and do away with the other provisions. For instance, it is not appropriate to treat the dependent exemption like a tax shelter, whereas it is appropriate to limit the use of private-purpose state and local bonds. There is no reason not to prohibit the exclusion of interest on these bonds within the regular income tax. Another way to keep the AMT in check over time is to raise its top rate and grant exemptions high enough to exclude most or all lower-, middle-, and upper-middle-income taxpayers. One way or the other, AMT reform as a whole is going to require a significant increase in either income tax rates or the tax base to keep revenues constant.

Tax All Capital Income Once

The notion that the combined corporate and individual income tax should tax all income once, and only once, at regular income tax rates, is sound. Once integrated, the corporate tax rate should be made equal to the top rate paid by individuals. In that way, most capital owners would not be led to choose the form of business, form of financing, and level of dividend payments on the basis of the tax system.[8]

Currently, a portion of corporate income is taxed at both the individual and the corporate levels (but at a maximum rate of 15 percent at the personal level), another portion is taxed at either the corporate or the individual level, and a final portion escapes taxation completely. Corporate income escapes taxation at the corporate level through shelters. It escapes taxation at the individual level to the extent that it accrues to nonprofits and pension funds. While the emphasis and public discussion has been on the so-called double-taxation of corporate income, the non-taxation—or sheltering—of corporate income is also a big problem.

Integrating the individual and corporate income taxes involves achieving several objectives that should be dealt with *simultaneously*. First, the creation of windfall gains should be minimized. Second, individual-level taxation of corporate dividends and capital gains should be waived only if the full tax has been paid on income at the corporate level.[9] If corporate taxes have not been paid, corporate dividends and real capital gains should be taxed at the *full* individual rate (not capped at 15 percent). Third, efforts to shut down corporate tax sheltering need to be substantially strengthened. Broadly defined, corporate sheltering occurs when firms engage in transactions that make sense only for tax reasons and do not have an underlying business purpose. Several examples involving the creative use of financial instruments have been well publicized in recent years. Although it is arguable whether such transactions are legal under current rules, our view is that the rules should be changed to either make such transactions illegal or make them unprofitable. This could be accomplished through increased enforcement as well as through the implementation of accounting procedures that require more conformity between book and taxable income. Fourth, corporate tax expenditures should be sharply curtailed. Corporate tax expenditures provide subsidies for investments in particular industries or activities, such as energy, manufacturing, and insurance. This package of changes would likely raise net federal revenues from corporate source income.[10]

Tax Labor Income Once

For about 75 percent of all households and virtually all wage earners in the bottom 40 percent of the income distribution, payroll tax burdens exceed income tax payments. The payroll tax imposes a burden of roughly 15 percent on the very first dollar of earnings.[11] In contrast, a family of four does not fall into the 15 percent marginal income tax bracket until its income exceeds $36,000 and does not pay an average 15 percent income tax rate until its income is $120,000, which is actually higher than the payroll tax cap for Social Security. Integrating the payroll tax and the income tax could take different forms, but could be done in a way that would make the burden of payroll taxes less regressive. This would be particularly important if a consumption tax either were added to the system or replaced part of the system, in order to offset some of the regressivity of such a tax.

Simplify

There are a number of ways to simplify the system, even without enacting massive reform. The administration's efforts to unify the definition of a child in the tax code is one such example. Movement toward return-free filing, or IRS completion of tax returns, could be achieved for as many as 50 million taxpayers in the United States, but would require some adjustments in the tax code. The number of households who could avoid filing would be greatly enhanced, and other simplifications would occur, if the personal exemption, the child credit, and the earned income credit were consolidated into a single program, and if the standard deduction were increased. Other areas ripe for simplification via consolidation involve education subsidies and retirement saving programs.

Improve Administration and Enforcement

Intelligent tax reform would equip the Internal Revenue Service with the resources it needs to enforce and administer the system. Many taxpayers simply do not pay the taxes they owe. Providing the IRS with additional resources to better enforce current tax rules would likely boost revenues by more than the cost of the additional resources. At the same time, one can only go so far in this direction before the costs exceed the benefits.

Raise Revenue Levels to Meet Government Spending Needs

Under plausible projections and with no significant entitlement reform, federal spending will rise to about 27 percent of GDP in the not-too-distant future (as described in chapter 2). Historically, revenues have stayed below 20 percent of GDP. If outlays are allowed to rise to such levels, or even to somewhat lower levels, serious thought needs to be given to how best to structure a tax system not only at current revenue levels, but also at the levels that those expenditures might require. To be clear, this is an argument for paying honestly for any chosen size of government, not an argument about what that size should be. If higher spending requires additional revenues, it will be even more important than it is now to keep rates as low as possible and the base as broad as possible, for purposes of achieving both efficiency and equity.

One possibility—at least, there is strong evidence that it can be administered—is a value added tax. A broad-based VAT, one with only a few exclusions, would generate revenue of about 0.6 percent of GDP for each percentage point of tax.[12] It would also affect prices, and thus increase the cost of government purchases and reduce the income tax base. The net contribution to deficit reduction, therefore, would be about 0.4 percent of GDP for each percentage point of tax. On balance, then, a 10 percent VAT could raise an additional 4 to 5 percent of GDP in revenue, if its tax base were kept fairly broad.

The great advantage of a VAT over a national retail sales tax is that the VAT is a proven collection system that is used in more than 100 countries around the world. Exporters could follow established procedures for getting rebates at the border. Unlike the retail sales tax, the VAT has certain features that allow it to effectively tax services as well as goods. Furthermore, one form of VAT uses credits that effectively reduce the amount of cheating by requiring users of inputs to make up for missing VAT if their suppliers have not paid them. Administrative concerns make the NRST a much more questionable proposition, even as a supplement to the existing system.

Another avenue of approach is to impose a tax on carbon emissions or establish a market in rights to emit carbon. These options would deal with a major environmental problem as well as contribute to revenues. Such taxes, however, are likely to raise far less in revenues than a moderate value added tax and also raise significant issues of environmental policy that are beyond the scope of this chapter.

Revenue Packages

Table 5-1 shows alternative ways of combining the ideas above to both meet various possible revenue goals and restructure taxes.

Structural Reforms

At any level of revenue, structural reforms would be desirable, including a no-return system for many households, restructured saving incentives, integration of corporate and individual income taxes, consolidation of

Table 5-1. *Financing Options for 2030*
Percent of GDP

Item	Smaller government scenario		Two intermediate government scenarios				Larger government scenario	
	1	2	3	4	5	6	7	8
Spending	18	18	24	24	24	24	28	28
Revenue[a]	20	20	20	20	20	20	20	20
Repeal AMT	–0.5	–0.5						
Cut rates	–1.5	–3.5						
Allow tax cuts to expire			2	2			2	
Aggressively reduce tax expenditures		2	2		2		2	
5% VAT				2	2			
10% VAT						4	4	
20% VAT								8
Total revenue	18	18	24	24	24	24	28	28

Source: Authors' calculations, as discussed in text.
a. In adjusted baseline.

existing programs for education and for saving, and consolidation of the earned income, child credit, and personal exemption. In addition, a thorough cleaning of the tax base, featuring a substantial trimming of tax expenditures, would be in order. Whether the revenues obtained from base broadening or other measures are used to raise overall revenues or reduce tax rates across the board will depend on the level of government spending.

Revenues to Finance the Smaller Government Scenario

The adjusted baseline makes the 2001 and 2003 tax cuts permanent, indexes the AMT for inflation, and no longer treats the dependent exemption like a tax shelter for AMT purposes. Under the smaller government scenario described in chapter 2, federal spending is 18.2 percent of GDP by 2030. Still, this is *lower* than revenues under the adjusted baseline, which would be 20 percent of GDP in that year.[13] The "excess" revenue would allow policymakers to move the antisheltering provisions of the AMT into the regular income tax and then repeal the AMT altogether. It would also allow additional rate cuts.

Revenues to Finance the Two Intermediate Scenarios

Under the two intermediate scenarios discussed in chapter 2, investing in the future and maintaining the social contract, spending is about 24 percent of GDP by 2030, roughly 4 percent of GDP above the adjusted revenue baseline. This difference could be closed through several changes. Allowing the tax cuts to expire would raise 2 percent of GDP in revenue. A 5 (or 10) percent VAT would raise about 2 (or 4) percent of GDP in revenue. Aggressive closing of tax expenditures could raise another 1 to 2 percent of GDP in revenue (if the revenues were not used to reduce rates). Note that the cost of making the 2001 and 2003 tax cuts permanent is roughly equivalent to an extra 5 percentage points on the value added tax.

Another possibility—that we do not pursue here—would be an additional mandate on individuals to pay for health and retirement programs, which could be assessed in ways other than a Social Security tax or a VAT. For example, individuals could be required to make deposits into retirement accounts and contribute toward their own retirement health insurance.

Revenues to Finance the Larger Government Scenario

In the larger government plan, spending would equal 28 percent of GDP in 2030, 8 percentage points above the adjusted revenue baseline. Under this scenario, allowing the tax cuts to expire, trimming a net of 2 percent of GDP in tax expenditures (using any excess to reduce tax rates), and implementing a value added tax of 10 percent would all be required to match the increase in government spending. If tax expenditures could not be trimmed and the tax cuts were made permanent, a 20 percent VAT would be required to balance the budget.

Conclusion

The structure of the tax system should be improved regardless of the level of government spending. Cutting back on tax subsidies performs the same economic function as cutting back on direct expenditures and permits a lowering of the tax rates required to support government. But revenue increases will also be required, unless policymakers are willing to keep spending below the adjusted baseline, particularly in the areas of health and retirement.

Notes

1. Due to length restrictions, we necessarily omit many important issues that a fuller treatment would permit. For more detailed discussions of our views, see Henry J. Aaron, William Gale, and James Sly, "The Rocky Road to Tax Reform," in *Setting National Priorities: The 2000 Election and Beyond,* edited by Henry J. Aaron and Robert D. Reischauer (Brookings, 1999), pp. 211–66; William Gale and Janet Holtzblatt, "The Role of Administrative Issues in Tax Reform: Simplicity, Compliance, and Administration," in *United States Tax Reform in the Twenty-First Century,* edited by George R. Zodrow and Peter Mieszkowski (Cambridge University Press, 2002), pp. 179–214; and C. Eugene Steuerle, "Tax Reform: Prospects and Possibilities," statement before the Committee on the Budget, U.S. House of Representatives, October 6, 2004.

2. A key exception to this statement is the case of "externalities," such as pollution, where the activity of one person or group imposes costs for other groups that are not borne by the original group.

3. For a recent analysis, see Robert Dennis and others, "Macroeconomic Analysis of a 10% Cut in Income Tax Rates," Technical Paper Series (Washington: Congressional Budget Office, May 2004). Similar analysis applies to federal spending programs as well. The programs have direct effects on household and business income and incentives, and if they are not financed by other spending cuts or tax increases they increase budget deficits, which exerts a drag on long-term economic activity.

4. Robert E. Hall and Alvin Rabushka, *The Flat Tax* (Stanford, Calif.: Hoover Institution Press, 1995).

5. Another consumption tax alternative is the USA (unified saving account) tax; see Laurence S. Seidman, *The USA Tax: A Progressive Consumption Tax* (MIT Press, 1997). This proposal would combine a VAT on businesses with a personal consumption tax. Under the personal tax, people would report all income from earnings, investments, and receipt of loans, but they would be allowed a new deduction for all net saving and repayment of loans. Thus, the personal tax falls on the difference between income and saving, which is consumption. In addition, the USA tax would retain some of the deductions and credits allowed under the current personal income tax and would have progressive rates. The USA tax has been judged to have large administrative problems, partly because of the attempt to retain the existing progressivity of the income tax.

6. Official estimates of many subsidies are contained in a tax expenditure budget prepared each year by the Tax Department. See Office of Management and

Budget, "Tax Expenditures," in *Fiscal Year 2006, Analytical Perspectives, Budget of the U.S. Government* (Government Printing Office, 2005).

7. A similar story could be also told about many direct spending programs—farm subsidies come to mind.

8. Similarly, with this integration, there should be only one corporate tax rate. We see no reason to assess lower taxes on rich owners of corporate capital than more modest owners simply because the latter's shares happen to be in a larger corporation.

9. If corporate taxes had been paid, an alternative to taxing corporate source income at a zero rate at the personal level would be to provide a credit at the personal level. This would allow corporate source income to be taxed on a personalized basis, so that low-income households do not bear the full 35 percent rate.

10. The comprehensive business income tax (CBIT) proposal offered by the Treasury Department in 1992 would eliminate interest deductions for firms and exclude dividends and interest from individual taxation, and would apply to unincorporated businesses as well as corporations. This proposal also affects the returns to old capital, however, not just new capital.

11. The available evidence suggests that workers bear the burden, via reduced wages, of both their own payroll tax payments and those made by their employer. See Harvey S. Rosen, *Public Finance*, 6th ed. (New York: McGraw-Hill/Irwin, 2001), pp. 265–66.

12. Henry J. Aaron, William G. Gale, and Peter R. Orszag, "Meeting the Revenue Challenge," in *Restoring Fiscal Sanity: How to Balance the Budget*, edited by Alice M. Rivlin and Isabel Sawhill (Brookings, 2004), p. 122.

13. The main reason revenues rise as a share of GDP in the adjusted baseline is that under current law, brackets in the regular income tax and the AMT are not indexed for real wage growth (only for inflation), so that over time productivity growth would push people into higher tax brackets.

6

The Politics of Deficit Reduction

ISABEL SAWHILL AND
RON HASKINS

Addressing the fiscal challenges facing the country in 2005 and beyond is daunting. Fundamental disagreements exist about what government should do and how to pay for it. Most Democrats are eager to preserve Social Security and Medicare more or less intact, as well as to protect the social safety net for low-income families and a host of other programs that are a legacy of the New Deal and the Great Society. Most Republicans, on the other hand, would like to keep tax rates low, limit the size and scope of government, and return to individuals more responsibility to provide for their own welfare, health care, and retirement. Neither party wants to adversely affect their constituents by either cutting spending or raising taxes for fear of retribution at the polls. Yet the fiscal challenge cannot be met unless a way is found to deal with these disagreements and barriers to action.

We are deeply indebted to Steve Robblee and Daniel Klaff for their extensive assistance with this chapter. We would also like to acknowledge the participation of the twenty interview subjects and thank them for their time and interesting comments.

In this chapter we address the substantial political challenge associated with restoring fiscal responsibility. As difficult as it may be, the nation must meet this challenge head-on for all of the reasons cited in earlier chapters. We begin with a brief history of efforts to pass legislation to reduce budget deficits or reform taxes. We then distill from this history and from insights drawn from students of American government a number of lessons that might help guide any new effort to close the gap between spending and revenues. Finally, we report on interviews with twenty budget experts who are, or have been, involved in negotiating budget agreements or related legislation. These interviews provide insight into the factors that shape budget negotiations and the prospects for significant deficit reduction over the next few years.

A Look Backward

A brief review of earlier agreements provides a set of case studies that illuminates both the barriers to greater fiscal responsibility and the ways in which those barriers have been overcome in the past. Specifically, we review the Social Security reforms of 1983, the tax reforms of 1986, and the budget agreements of 1990, 1993, and 1997.

1983 Social Security Reforms

The Social Security system faced insolvency in 1981 that would, if not fixed before July 1983, threaten to delay the full benefit checks of 36 million Americans.[1] To buy time and propose solutions, President Reagan established a fifteen member bipartisan commission with Alan Greenspan at its helm.[2] The commission recommended and Congress adopted a number of measures that not only solved the short-term problem of insolvency, but also improved the financing problem over the medium term. The most important of these measures were an increase in the Social Security payroll tax, a deferral of the annual cost-of-living adjustment for one quarter, a new tax on Social Security benefits received by upper-income participants, and the extension of coverage to most workers previously excluded (federal and nonprofit employees).

The independent commission's suggestions made up two-thirds of the seventy-five-year funding shortfall. As the bill worked its way through Congress, Representative Jake Pickle, a senior Democrat on the House Ways and Means Committee, after considerable behind-the-scenes work with colleagues on both sides of the aisle, offered a successful floor amendment to gradually raise the age at which full benefits could be received from sixty-five to sixty-seven, beginning in 2003. The final legislation was signed into law on April 20, 1983.

The success of this effort was due in part to the use of an independent commission, which provided political cover for the president and Congress while they considered changes to a highly popular program. In addition, the public perceived the mix of tax increases and benefit reductions as distributing the pain broadly. Finally, the public was willing to consider changes to Social Security because the program's financial viability appeared to be in imminent danger.

1986 Tax Reforms

In his 1984 State of the Union address, President Reagan promised "to simplify the entire tax code so all taxpayers, big and small, are treated more fairly."[3] Almost three years later, on October 22, he signed the Tax Reform Act of 1986. Broadly characterized, the final bill shifted part of the tax burden from individuals to corporations, broadened the base of taxable income by eliminating many loopholes (deductions and credits), and lowered tax rates on both individuals and corporations. Most households received a tax cut and 6 million poor people were removed from the tax rolls entirely. The top rate on individuals plummeted from 50 percent to 33 percent, while the top corporate rate fell from 48 percent to 34 percent.[4]

Several factors played a part in the success of this legislation. These included presidential leadership; bipartisan support from key members of Congress; a public consensus that the tax system was too complicated and unfair; and political considerations—neither party wanted to be accused of blocking tax reform in the run-up to the 1986 midterm elections. It is especially notable that both parties gave up something to gain something. Democrats accepted lower rates on wealthy taxpayers, but achieved the complete elimination of federal income taxes on millions of low-income families; Republicans accepted a greater tax burden on corporations to reduce the tax burden on the wealthy and the middle class. This willingness of both parties to compromise produced legislation that economists hailed as fulfilling their traditional admonition to promote equity and efficiency by broadening the tax base while reducing rates.

Unfortunately, once the legislation was passed, the process of lobbying for tax benefits began anew. Many of the loopholes closed in 1986 have been reopened, and new ones have been added to the law.

1990 Budget Act

From the end of World War II until Reagan was elected in 1980, federal deficits were not a major problem. They tended to increase during periods of recession and subside once the economy recovered (figure 6-1). But the tax cuts enacted on a bipartisan basis in 1981 along with the large increases in defense spending that were part of the "Reagan revolution" reshaped the fiscal landscape, producing unprecedented peacetime deficits. Congress and President Reagan reacted by enacting tax increases that reversed some of the revenue losses of 1981 and by passing the Balanced Budget and Emergency Deficit Control Act of 1985, better known as "Gramm-Rudman-Hollings" (GRH). GRH proved incapable of forcing the needed budgetary discipline because it focused on total deficits, which are heavily influenced by economic and technical assumptions beyond the control of Congress, and because Congress proved adept at procedural maneuvers designed to subvert the GRH controls. In July 1990, the Congressional Budget Office projected a sharp increase in the fiscal 1991 budget deficit. GRH rules called for draconian spending cuts that were substantively indefensible and politically infeasible. Something else had to be done.

That something was the Omnibus Budget Reconciliation Act of 1990 (OBRA1990). The new law grew out of a long and difficult budget summit. Democrats had a comfortable majority in both houses, but not enough to overcome a veto. Thus, cooperation with President George H. W. Bush was essential. He signaled his willingness to consider tax increases as part of the deal, despite his memorable campaign commitment to "no new taxes." The parties agreed to conduct a summit with

Figure 6-1. *Deficits as a Proportion of the U.S. Economy, 1950–2004*

Deficit or surplus (percent GDP)

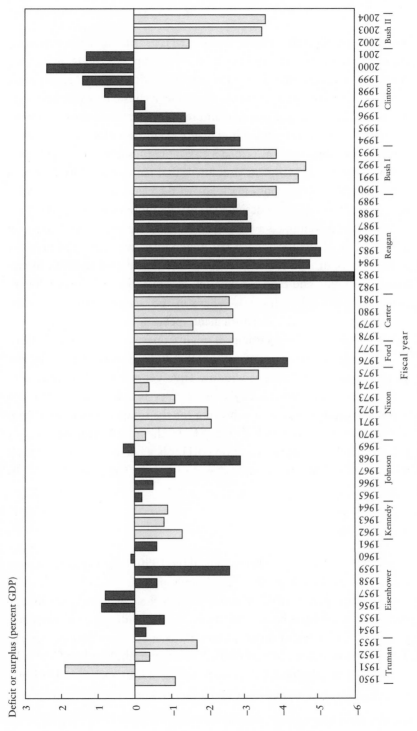

Fiscal year

Source: *Budget of the U.S. Government*, Fiscal Year 2006 Historical Tables (Government Printing Office, 2005), table 1.2.

seventeen members, three from the White House and fourteen represent-
ing both parties in Congress. But even this group was too large and too
divided to reach an accord and was later pared down to just eight people
who hammered out an agreement.[5] Revealing a chasm between their posi-
tion on tax increases and that of their president, a large majority of House
Republicans voted against the initial agreement, resulting in its defeat. It
was not until the president vetoed a continuing resolution on October 6,
causing a partial government shutdown, that Congress finally enacted a
reconciliation bill incorporating many of the elements of the agreement
plus several new elements designed to attract more Democratic votes.

OBRA1990 contained a package of tax and spending measures projected to reduce the deficit by $482 billion over five years. The new law
included a Budget Enforcement Act (BEA) that placed caps on discretionary spending and required that any new tax cuts or increases in entitlement spending be offset elsewhere in the budget through revenue
increases or reductions in entitlement spending (this requirement was
called "PAYGO"). By focusing on what Congress could control (legislated changes in spending and taxes rather than the total deficit), by creating a longer-term budget window (five years instead of one) with
enforcement every year, and by viewing rules as a way to preserve past
agreements rather than as a substitute for the tough substantive actions
needed to reduce large pre-existing deficits, these BEA rules were widely
perceived to be an improvement on GRH. They played an important role
in reducing deficits in the 1990s.[6] Unfortunately, Congress allowed the
rules to expire in 2002.

1993 Budget Act

A recession in the early 1990s prevented the 1990 budget agreement from
reducing the deficit as much as had been hoped. In the 1992 presidential
election, Ross Perot talked incessantly about the deficit and won enough
votes to put the issue back onto the national agenda. Thus it is not surprising that, after winning the election, President Clinton decided to make
deficit reduction a major part of his economic program.

His deficit reduction package was enacted in the summer of 1993 by a
vote of 218 to 216 in the House and a tie-breaking vote by Vice President

Gore in the Senate. The package received no Republican support and even some Democrats rejected it. Even so, it was estimated to reduce the deficit by $433 billion over five years by virtually freezing discretionary spending (in nominal terms) and by raising taxes, primarily on the wealthy.[7]

Unlike earlier legislation, this law was a purely partisan affair in which the president took advantage of the Democratic majority in both houses to enact his program. Much as Bush had paid a price at the polls in 1992 for reneging on his "no new taxes" pledge, Democrats in the House later paid a price for the tax increases that were a major part of their deficit-reducing efforts. Combined with scandals in the House and the defeat of Clinton's health plan, the tax increases played a role in a devastating reversal of the Democrats' political fortunes in the 1994 midterm elections. The clear lesson is that the political risks associated with tackling a deficit loom very large. But the risks to the economy of doing nothing are also large, creating a real dilemma for the political party in power.

1997 Budget Act

The 1994 election gave the Republican Party both chambers of Congress for a full congressional term for the first time since 1932. By June 1995 Republicans had enacted a budget resolution that would have balanced the budget within seven years while cutting taxes by $245 billion. Spending cuts totaled $894 billion and included steep cuts of $450 billion in Medicare and Medicaid over this seven-year period.[8]

A group of conservative House Democrats wrote a compromise bill designed to attract more Democratic support. The compromise bill would have balanced the budget without cutting taxes—following the principle that tax cuts should not come before a balanced budget.[9] However, the Republican-led Congress ignored the compromise proposal and passed a bill, with little support from Democrats, closely mirroring their original budget resolution. Clinton, as promised, vetoed the Republican bill, setting off a major confrontation over the budget. Political stalemate between Clinton and congressional Republicans continued throughout the fall, winter, and early spring. A series of short-term spending agreements called "continuing resolutions" allowed the government to operate without a budget during much of this period, but the federal government was partially shut down on two separate occasions for a total of twenty-seven days.[10] The two sides did not reach agreement on a budget until April 25, 1996, nearly seven months after the fiscal year began.

The 1997 budget agreement was forged with less partisan bickering than the highly fractious debates of 1995 and 1996. The Republican-controlled Congress and the White House first agreed on a set of goals for the 1997 budget package and then negotiated a path to get there. To achieve the goal of a balanced budget by 2002, Republicans and President Clinton set a target for deficit reduction that included roughly $350 billion in spending cuts and $85 billion in tax cuts over the five-year period.[11] Unexpectedly high economic growth produced higher revenues, allowing the final deficit reduction package to reduce spending by "only" $198 billion, including $119 billion in Medicare and Medicaid cuts, while still leaving room for an $81 billion tax cut.[12] The net effect of the bill was to reduce the deficit by $118 billion over the five-year period, 1998 to 2002.

Lessons Learned

As this brief history shows, the political barriers to deficit reduction have always been high. Any president or member of Congress that takes the steps needed to restore fiscal discipline may well suffer at the polls. Creating deficits by handing out tax cuts or benefit increases to the public is all pleasure; reducing them later brings pain. And even though the public at large would benefit from an agreement to reduce the deficit, specific groups would not. For members of Congress, political survival often depends on not offending such groups—whether they be the elderly, farmers, steel producers, wealthy individuals, or a myriad of other influential constituencies and their lobbying organizations that have vast resources at their disposal to fight spending cuts or tax increases.[13]

Some argue that deficits are not necessarily bad for the country because a deficit can crimp the ability of Congress or the president to increase spending. Over the past twenty years, however, reductions in taxes have gone hand in hand with increases in spending as a proportion of GDP, not the reverse.[14] Increasingly, members of Congress who have been the most committed to tax reductions, as shown by their willingness to sign a "no new taxes" pledge, have shown less concern for restraining spending.[15] One possible interpretation of this perverse result is that earlier norms about the importance of fiscal responsibility have eroded badly while the view that "deficits don't matter" has gained currency.

Given the difficulties of achieving deficit reduction, what might make it possible for elected officials to act in more fiscally responsible ways? The history of prior efforts to deal with contentious budgetary and tax issues, together with academic research, suggests a number of lessons that may prove instructive in addressing the current deficit.

Lesson One: The Public Must Demand Action

Elected officials may not take the painful steps required to reduce the deficit unless the public demands that something be done. Yet there is little likelihood of public outcry until members of the public become educated and concerned about the issue. The public will be apathetic if its leaders are not talking about the problem, and confused if these leaders disagree about the deficit's importance. Early introduction of the issue into the national conversation is crucial because there may be a lag between the time policy experts recognize the problem and the time its seriousness begins to affect popular opinion. Perhaps most importantly, in the absence of strong evidence that deficits are affecting their lives, members of the public may not become sufficiently energized to insist on tough remedies. In 2004 a little more than 50 percent of the public ranked the deficit as a top priority, up from 35 percent in 2002. But this is still lower than the 65 percent of the public that ranked the deficit as a top priority in late 1994.[16] Many observers believe it will take some kind of economic crisis to catalyze public opinion behind serious efforts to reduce the deficit.

Lesson Two: Presidential Leadership Is Important

Even with an economic crisis, and certainly in its absence, a president's ability to set the agenda and to spend political capital on his main priorities are important ingredients in major budget legislation. In his first term, President George W. Bush seemed less concerned about the deficit than his predecessors. He supported the establishment of a new and expensive entitlement to prescription drugs for the elderly; he reduced federal revenues to their lowest percentage of GDP since 1950; and he did not veto a single spending bill. In his second term, Bush has pledged more restraint in nondefense discretionary spending and has backed Social Security changes that would increase personal investment and eventually cut promised benefits, but only after adding more than $4 trillion to deficits over the first two decades these proposals are in effect.[17] He also favors extending tax cuts that would greatly reduce revenues over the next decade and beyond and supports a growth rate in military spending that exceeds inflation. These positions have left many observers skeptical of the president's willingness to lead the very painful fight that will be necessary to reduce the deficit.

Lessons one and two often work together. Jonathan Rauch of the *National Journal* has argued that two things are necessary to change a policy supported by narrow, short-term interests that conflict with the long-term welfare of the nation. The first is a public that believes an important problem exists whose solution will produce a "collective payoff." The second is a leader with the vision to create effective reforms and the political skills to get them enacted.[18] At this point, the public is only moderately concerned about the deficit, although its concern is growing, and no senior elected official, including the president, has stepped up to propose a deficit reduction plan and then lead the fight necessary to enact it.

Lesson Three: Bipartisanship Works Best

At first glance, one-party government—in which the same party controls the White House and Congress—would seem to increase the chances of passing legislation to improve the long-term budget outlook. After all, with single-party control, the House or Senate is less likely to block a bill passed by the other chamber, and the president is less likely to veto a bill passed by Congress. But divisions between the two houses can be sharp and academic research into the relationship between one-party control of Congress and the presidency and the passage of legislation is mixed. Some researchers argue that one-party control eases the passage of legislation, while others hold that it does not.[19]

Whatever legislative success is achieved in a one-party system, it may be short-lived if it has little or no support from the minority that is out of power. The first five chapters of this volume—not to mention numerous other books and analyses from the Congressional Budget Office (CBO) and the Government Accountability Office (GAO)—argue that solving the deficit problem will require very tough decisions about the long-term structure of tax and entitlement programs. Changes must not only gain acceptance in the present, but must have staying power for many years or even decades. An agreement founded on principles acceptable to both mainstream Republicans and Democrats is more likely to hold up over time.[20]

The budget deal of 1993 shows what can happen when the interests of the minority are excluded. The Clinton 1993 tax increase, primarily affecting the affluent, was partially reversed by the Bush 2001 tax cut. By contrast, PAYGO rules and discretionary spending caps were created under a bipartisan agreement in 1990 and were reaffirmed through two extensions (in 1993 and 1997) before dying in 2002 under a one-party government that saw budget restrictions as a hindrance to achieving other tax and spending objectives. As a former budget director we interviewed, who has been involved in numerous budget negotiations, said, "I have done it both ways, and I prefer bipartisan."

Lesson Four: Everything Should Be on the Table

Previous chapters showed that the long-term deficit problem is so great that there is no one solution that will bring projected budgets into balance. Raising taxes or cutting spending alone will not solve the problem. Nor can the nation simply grow its way out of deficits because the costs of health care and Social Security for the elderly are increasing faster than any plausible projection of economic growth. Under these circumstances, all policy options should be on the table. Eliminating any broad policy avenue from consideration—raising taxes, cutting discretionary spending, curtailing entitlements—makes the job of restoring fiscal sanity virtually impossible.

Putting everything on the table is a necessity not only because the problem is large, but also because to achieve lasting consensus the pain must be spread broadly. The best hope of assembling a congressional majority in favor of taking decisive action on the deficit is to create a compromise that inflicts pain on both sides. Generally, this means that Republicans must agree to tax increases while Democrats agree to spending cuts.

Lesson Five: Unorthodox Methods of Legislating Can Help

Another potential mechanism for avoiding some of the problems inherent in congressional action on budget deficits involves using unorthodox methods of legislating that provide political cover for members of Congress.[21] For the longer term, more thought should be given to needed reforms in political institutions themselves—an important topic, but one that goes beyond the scope of this chapter.

The Social Security Commission of 1982 and the budget summit of 1990 provide examples of how Congress can delegate difficult decisions to extra-legal bodies. Legislation in the late 1980s and 1990s that sought to close military bases provides another example.[22] A final example is so-called "fast-track" trade authority, which gives presidents the power to negotiate international trade agreements that are voted on by Congress, but cannot be amended.

President Bush has already used two commissions to further his own legislative agenda. In 2002 he appointed a commission to make recommendations on Social Security reform that may heavily influence the administration's own proposal. Similarly, the president has appointed a commission to make recommendations about tax reform that he will presumably use to fashion his own proposal in the next year or two. These commissions are models of trying to build support for policy proposals that later form the basis of specific legislation. If the president or Congress were to appoint a bipartisan commission to recommend steps to reduce the budget deficit, the commission's work could form the basis for legislation that might address all the elements of an eventual bipartisan compromise: Social Security, Medicare and Medicaid, taxes, and other spending.

Lesson Six: Rules Matter

Under Senate rules, any senator can filibuster a given bill and a group of senators can filibuster indefinitely by taking turns on the Senate floor. The only way to stop a filibuster is to hold a vote to close debate that garners at least sixty votes. In effect, the rules governing filibusters mean that the majority party must have sixty votes to pass major legislation.

Reconciliation bills, however, cannot be filibustered. Reconciliation is a part of the congressional budget process and depends on the adoption of a congressional budget resolution or plan that spells out spending, revenue, and deficit targets for a five- or ten-year period, with reconciliation instructions. These instructions require certain committees to approve measures that cut mandatory spending or raise revenues by set amounts. These measures are then assembled into one or more omnibus reconciliation bills.

During the 1990s, reconciliation bills were often used to reduce the deficit. Special budget rules requiring sixty votes in the Senate on any tax or mandatory spending measure that was not paid for or that exceeded legislated caps on discretionary spending greatly aided the deficit reduction process. As noted earlier, these PAYGO rules and caps proved to be an effective way of maintaining fiscal discipline in the 1990s. However, even PAYGO and spending caps were violated by Congress once surpluses developed after 1997; these rules were officially abandoned in 2002.

Bush has advocated renewing these rules in modified form. His proposal—which was introduced in 2004 as the Spending Control Act—would limit increases in discretionary spending and would re-institute PAYGO for mandatory spending legislation.[23] The law would not require offsets for tax cuts, however. For this reason it has been fiercely resisted by most Democrats and some moderate Republicans who argue that fiscal discipline requires holding the line on taxes as well as on spending.

One approach that has been advocated by some as a means of maintaining budget discipline is to give the president more authority to eliminate individual spending or tax provisions from multipart bills through a line-item veto or an enhanced rescission authority. In 1996 the Republican Congress passed the Line Item Veto Act, which allowed the president to veto specific spending items in large, omnibus bills that often contain hundreds or thousands of provisions. The line-item veto would allow presidents to veto certain individual expenditures in the annual appropriation and authorizing bills and could be overridden only by a two-thirds vote of both houses of Congress. When Clinton attempted to use this new line-item veto power, his rescissions were challenged and found to be unconstitutional by the Supreme Court.[24] Nonetheless, many experts believe a law could be written to avoid this constitutional problem by giving the president the power to propose a package of spending cuts that would have to be considered by Congress under streamlined procedures, including a fixed period of time, no amendments, and no filibuster in the Senate.

Last year's volume of *Restoring Fiscal Sanity* discussed these budget rules in more detail and argued that such rules can help Congress do the right thing by shifting blame from individual members to the rules themselves. Specifically, reinstating PAYGO for both mandatory spending and taxes, together with discretionary caps over a multiyear period, would be desirable. In addition, Congress should not be allowed to enact tax and mandatory spending laws that expire as a way of hiding their true costs. Finally, limiting what is considered to be "emergency spending" and developing better ways of measuring and highlighting longer-term budgetary commitments would also be desirable.

What Expert Observers of the Process Say

To understand more about the factors that influenced major compromise agreements, and to develop insights about how these factors might apply to our current budget predicament, we interviewed twenty Washington insiders. Half were Democrats and half Republicans; all had participated directly (as one of the principals) or indirectly (as a staff member of a principal) in formulating one or more of the agreements examined in this chapter.

We asked these experts to discuss, based on their experience, the importance of several factors in achieving the compromise agreements. The factors we identified included presidential leadership, one-party government, bipartisanship, use of nonofficial processes such as commissions and secret negotiations, external threats such as a financial crisis, and congressional budget processes or rules. We also asked the experts to rate the probability ("not likely," "somewhat likely," "very likely") that a budget deal and major reforms of the tax code, Social Security, and Medicare would be achieved in the next several years.

Sixteen of the twenty respondents mentioned external factors and presidential leadership as important in achieving a budget compromise. Bipartisanship was mentioned by thirteen of the respondents. Other factors mentioned, but only by two or three of the respondents, were a perception by both sides that the agreement was fair, a long and serious debate about the problem that produced some consensus, and an aroused public. A one-party government, use of nonofficial processes, and congressional rules were hardly mentioned at all. Generalizing across the views of these experienced experts in budget compromise and applying them to our current impasse, we conclude that an external threat, presidential leadership, and bipartisanship are the most important factors that could help forge a budget compromise.

These experts were also in substantial agreement about the prospects for a major budget deal and for Medicare reform. In both cases, sixteen of the twenty respondents said an agreement was not likely. A pervasive belief, among both Republicans and Democrats, that Republicans would not agree to tax increases was the primary reason our respondents felt a budget deal was unlikely.

There was slightly greater optimism about the prospects for reform of taxes, with eight of the twenty rating the likelihood of reform as somewhat likely and one as very likely. However, most respondents stated that only modest tax reforms could be passed, although Republicans pushing the reforms would likely try to make it appear that the reforms were major. One respondent, a former Republican senior staffer, reflected the views of many others when he said that Republicans "will change the definition of tax reform [by passing] modest changes like loophole closing and call[ing] it tax reform."

Social Security was the one program that a majority of our budget experts believed had a decent chance of being reformed. Twelve of the nineteen respondents (one declined to respond) thought it "very" or "somewhat" likely. Reading their comments makes it clear that most thought reform would be based on some type of private account. The major reason respondents gave for their optimism about Social Security reform was President Bush's determination to push reform.

In designing our questionnaire, we assumed that these experts would likely rate the prospects for Republican support of tax increases as low.

But Republicans might at least make progress on deficit reduction if they were determined to cut spending. Thus, we asked respondents to speculate on how much Congress could reduce spending relative to the CBO baseline. Fifteen of the twenty respondents said 1 percent or less, and only one thought spending could be cut by as much as 5 percent—and this only if there were a crisis such as a meltdown in the financial markets.

Clearly, Washington insiders think it unlikely that a major budget deal will pass in the near future. Nor is there any mystery about why they reach this conclusion. Given that most of our respondents believed that a major compromise would need to be bipartisan and involve both tax increases and spending cuts, the stance on taxes by the president and Congress virtually eliminates the prospect of a major budget deal. Thus, to the extent that the deficit is to be reduced over the next several years, it appears that Republicans will have to do it themselves and that it will involve only spending cuts. But given that hardly anyone thinks spending can be cut by more than 1 percent relative to the CBO baseline, serious progress against the deficit does not appear to be in the cards.

An especially revealing outcome of the interviews was the general sense that Republicans, who control both houses of Congress and the presidency, show little inclination to address the deficit. As one of the respondents observed, this lack of commitment to attacking the deficit contrasts sharply with Republican fervor over deficit reduction when they first took over Congress in 1995. As some of our respondents noted, many Republicans now value tax cuts more than deficit reduction or agree with Vice President Cheney's claim that deficits don't matter. For whatever reason, with quite a few notable exceptions, the traditional Republican commitment to a balanced federal budget seems to have weakened.

Conclusion

The nation faces a budget deficit of historic proportions. The current deficit will join forces with the retirement of the baby boom generation beginning a few years from now. The resulting explosion of Social Security and especially Medicare spending, combined with inadequate revenues to support current commitments, will create a torrent of red ink. This scenario makes it unreasonable to continue on our present course.

And yet, that is precisely what seems to be in prospect for the next several years. There was striking agreement among the experts we interviewed that three factors are important in shaping major budget and budget-related deals: presidential leadership, bipartisanship, and an external threat to the federal budget or the economy. The importance of these same three factors was also evident in the case studies reviewed at the beginning of this chapter. If these three factors were in play, the president might be able to work with congressional leadership on a bipartisan basis to craft an agreement that reduced the budget deficit by some specified amount over five years. It would help if, going into negotiations, there were an understanding that the final deal would achieve its total deficit reduction by putting everything on the table—all revenues and all types of spending. If the president and senior members of both parties in Congress emphasized the threat to our economy posed by the deficit, and especially if they emphasized that Americans are living high on the hog now and leaving the bills to be paid by their children and grandchildren, the public would in all probability respond, as it did in the 1990s, by supporting tougher measures.

Stronger procedural rules would help Congress hew to the deficit-reduction path, but it takes a Congress committed to deficit reduction to institute these rules in the first place. In the end, the public gets the government it deserves. Although opinion polls suggest that public concern with the deficit is growing, it has not yet reached the level of the late 1980s or the mid-1990s when Congress and the president took several efficacious steps to reduce the deficit. Unless leaders in the private sector become sufficiently concerned about the actual or possible impact of large deficits on the economy and convince elected officials to act, the evidence presented in this chapter suggests that the nation is not going to reverse its fiscal course any time soon.

Notes

1. Timothy Clark, "Congress Avoiding Political Abyss by Approving Social Security Changes," *National Journal*, March 19, 1983, pp. 611–15.

2. Steven R. Weisman, "Preparing for Compromise but Refusing to Concede," *New York Times*, November 7, 1982, sec. 4, p. 1.

3. David E. Rosenbaum, "The Tax Reform Act of 1986: How the Measure Came Together; A Tax Bill for the Textbook," *New York Times*, October 23, 1986, p. D16.

4. Jeffrey H. Birnbaum and Alan S. Murray, *Showdown at Gucci Gulch: Lawmakers, Lobbyists, and the Unlikely Triumph of Tax Reform* (New York: Random House, 1987), Appendixes A and B.

5. This smaller group excluded Lloyd Bentsen and Dan Rostenkowski—the chairmen of the Senate and House tax-writing committees, respectively—and tax-increase opponent Newt Gingrich. The eight who remained were Nicholas Brady, secretary of the treasury; Richard Darman, director of the Office of Management and Budget; John Sununu, White House chief of staff; Representative Thomas Foley, Speaker of the House; Representative Richard Gephardt, majority leader; Representative Robert Michel, minority leader; Senator Bob Dole, minority leader; and Senator George Mitchell, majority leader. See Daniel P. Franklin, *Making Ends Meet* (Washington: CQ Press, 1993), p. 66–67, and Susan F. Rasky, "Capital Gains and Circles within Inner Circles: Behind the Budget Accord," *New York Times*, October 2, 1990, p. A22.

6. Though deficits increased in the early 1990s, they would have increased even faster without the spending curbs imposed by the BEA, the General Accounting Office (now Government Accountability Office) found. See GAO, "Budget Process: Issues concerning the 1990 Reconciliation Act," October 1994.

7. CBO, "The Economic and Budget Outlook: An Update," September 1993, table 2-2.

8. David E. Rosenbaum, "Congress Passes GOP Budget-Balancing Plan," *New York Times*, June 30, 1995, p. A1; and David Hess and Steven Thomma, "Congress OKs Deficit-Busting Plan," *Philadelphia Inquirer*, June 30, 1995, p. A1.

9. The *Washington Post*, among others, endorsed the compromise package, calling it "the best horse in the race thus far." See "A Good Budget Compromise," *Washington Post*, October 24, 1995, p. A16.

10. The government faced a partial government shutdown for six days between November 14, 1995, and November 20, 1995, and then again between December 15, 1995, and January 5, 1996. Six of the thirteen federal spending bills were signed by November 19, 1995. Spending bills that continued to be debated controlled functions such as defense, education, housing, and other social programs.

11. Eric Pianin, "Disagreements on Details of Budget Deal May Delay Congressional Action," *Washington Post*, May 14, 1997, p. A4.

12. CBO, "Economic and Budget Outlook: An Update," September 1997, tables 10 and 11.

13. James Q. Wilson, *American Government: Institutions and Politics* (Lexington, Mass.: D.C. Health and Company, 1980). From 1955 to 1999, the number of groups listed in the *Encyclopedia of Associations* rose from fewer than 5,000 to more than 20,000. By 1999, the K Street economy was at $1.45 billion, having grown by an average of 7.3 percent annually since 1997. In 1999, there were 14,205 lobbyist-client relationships and 12,113 active lobbyists in Washington. See Center for Responsive Politics, "Influence, Inc.: Summary," 2000 (www.opensecrets.org/pubs/lobby00/summary.asp).

14. See William A. Niskanen and Peter Van Doren, "Some Intriguing Findings about Federal Spending," paper prepared for the annual meeting of the Public Choice Society, Baltimore, Md., March 11–14, 2004; and William G. Gale and Brennan Kelly, "The 'No New Taxes' Pledge," *Tax Notes*, July 12, 2004, pp. 197–209.

15. More than half of the House of Representatives (222 of 435) and nearly half the Senate (42 of 100) have signed a "pledge" sponsored by Americans for Tax Reform vowing they will not increase income taxes. President Bush has also signed this pledge. Totals are as of December 13, 2004. See Americans for Tax Reform, "National Pledge" (www.atr.org/nationalpledge/index.html [December 13, 2004]).

16. The Pew Research Center for People and the Press conducted a poll five times between 1994 and 2004 using this question: "Should reducing the budget deficit be a top priority, important but lower priority, not too important, or should it not be done?" The percentage of people ranking the deficit a "top priority" were: 65 percent (December 1994), 60 percent (January 1997), 35 percent (January 2002), 40 percent (January 2003), and 51 percent (January 2004).

17. Peter R. Orszag, "Borrowing from Future Social Security Benefits: The Administration's Proposal for Individual Accounts," statement before the House Committee on the Budget, February 9, 2005.

18. Jonathan Rauch, *Government's End: Why Washington Stopped Working* (New York: Public Affairs, 1994), p. 198.

19. David R. Mayhew (in *Divided We Govern: Party Control, Lawmaking, and Investigations 1946-1990* [Yale University Press, 1991]) and Keith Krehbiel (in *Pivotal Politics: A Theory of U.S. Lawmaking* [University of Chicago Press, 1998]) are among those that find little or no benefit to one-party control. Sarah Binder has argued that one-party control and election mandates do matter empirically. Binder claims that a more complex model, which uses the percentage of agenda items that end in stalemate in each congressional session as the response variable, significantly alters the results found by Mayhew and others. See Sarah A. Binder, *Stalemate: Causes and Consequences of Legislative Gridlock* (Brookings, 2003).

20. Eric Patashnik, "After the Public Interest Prevails: The Political Sustainability of Policy Reform," *Governance* 16, no. 2 (2003): 203–234.

21. See Barbara Sinclair, *Unorthodox Lawmaking: New Legislative Processes in the U.S. Congress*, 2d ed. (Washington: CQ Press, 2000) and R. Kent Weaver, "The Politics of Blame Avoidance," *Journal of Public Policy* 6, no. 4 (1986): 371–398.

22. Four times between 1988 and 1995 Congress established an independent, bipartisan commission to close military bases. The process was integral to breaking a political stalemate that had inhibited base closings for three decades. The secretary of defense submitted a list of prospective bases to close with input from the military branches. The commission then held hearings, collected information, and modified the list. The commission's final list was then submitted to the president, who was able to either accept or reject the list as a whole. After presidential approval, the secretary of defense could begin closing bases unless Congress passed a joint resolution within 45 days to prevent all base closings. See Kenneth

R. Mayer, "Closing Military Bases (Finally): Solving Collective Dilemmas through Delegation," *Legislative Studies Quarterly* 20, no. 3 (1995): 393–413.

23. Spending limits for both discretionary and mandatory spending could be overridden by a three-fifths vote in the Senate. If the limits were exceeded, however, the Office of Management and Budget would be required to cut other non-exempt programs to make up the difference. See *Budget of the U.S. Government, Fiscal Year 2006* (Government Printing Office, 2005), pp. 26–27.

24. *Clinton* v. *City of New York*, 524 U.S. 417 (1998).

Contributors

HENRY J. AARON
Brookings Institution

WILLIAM G. GALE
Brookings Institution

RON HASKINS
Brookings Institution

JACK MEYER
Brookings Institution

PETER R. ORSZAG
Brookings Institution

RUDOLPH G. PENNER
Urban Institute

ALICE M. RIVLIN
Brookings Institution

ISABEL SAWHILL
Brookings Institution

JOHN B. SHOVEN
Stanford University

C. EUGENE STEUERLE
Urban Institute

Index

Aaron, Henry, 11–12
Advisory Council on Social Security
   (*1994–96*), 61
Afghanistan, 18, 29
Agency for International
   Development, 38
Aging. *See* Longevity
Agriculture, 36, 38, 49
AIME. *See* Average indexed monthly
   earnings
Alternative minimum tax (AMT). *See*
   Taxes and credits
Americans for Tax Reform, 137n15
AMT. *See* Alternative minimum tax
Asia, 5, 23
Average indexed monthly earnings
   (AIME), 68. *See also* Social
   Security

Baby boomers: Medicaid and, 83;
   population size, 25; retirement, 6,

35, 40, 58; Social Security and, 6,
   25, 60
Balanced Budget and Emergency
   Deficit Control Act of *1985*, 122,
   124
Bipartisanship, 128–30, 133
BEA. *See* Budget Enforcement Act
Belgium, 48–49
Budget. *See* Federal budget
Budget Act of *1993*, 124–25, 129
Budget Act of *1997*, 125–26
Budget Enforcement Act (BEA; *1990*),
   124
Bush, George H. W., 122, 124, 125
Bush, George W.: budget recommen-
   dations for *2006*, 21; concern
   about budget deficit, 127–28;
   reform of Social Security, 55, 57,
   133; Spending Control Act of
   2004, 131; tax cuts, 18; use of
   commissions, 130